DR. BERGER'S IMMUNE POWER DIET

by

Stuart M. Berger, M.D.

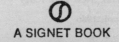

A SIGNET BOOK

NEW AMERICAN LIBRARY

A hardcover edition of *Dr. Berger's Immune Power Diet Plan* was
published by New American Library and simultaneously in Canada by
The New American Library of Canada Limited.

BREAK THE "IMMUNE-FAT CYCLE"

Take a good look at yourself: your body, your health, your emotional well-being. If you notice more than ½-inch of extra fat around your waistline . . . sudden binge-diet eating habits . . . low energy and stamina. . . mood swings . . . nasal congestion, headaches, stomach upsets, your excess weight may be causing an immune deficiency—which in turn makes it almost impossible for you to lose weight!

This uniquely effective nutritional program short-circuits that vicious cycle by eliminating the foods that disrupt your body's equilibrium. Without counting calories, the pounds and the symptoms disappear, for a lasting, positive change in not only *what you eat* but *how you feel*.

DR. BERGER'S IMMUNE POWER DIET

"NOT JUST A WEIGHT LOSS DIET . . . An interesting and systematic approach to tracking down food sensitivities . . . with appealing recipes and menus."

—*Publishers Weekly*

Ⓞ

Staying Healthy with SIGNET Books

Note to the Reader
The diet menus, charts, recipes, and guidelines contained in this work embody a practical application of the principles underlying the Immune Power Diet Plan. As in any other diet plan, you are urged to consult with your physician prior to commencing this diet program.

*This book is dedicated to my mother,
who, through diet and nutrition,
continues to win her battle against cancer.*

ACKNOWLEDGMENTS

There are five people who have made this book a reality and without any one of them its conception, organization, writing, and completion could not have happened. These five people are also some of my closest friends. In alphabetical order they are: Walter Anderson, Editor *Parade* Magazine, for his confidence; Lorna Darmour, the person responsible for my life; Oscar Dystel, a publishing genius; Scott Meredith, my super agent; and David Nimmons, who has done the actual writing and is responsible for translating many complicated ideas into English.

I express my gratitude to New American Library for its confidence in the concepts contained in the book and in the author. My special appreciation to Michaela Hamilton, Bob Diforio, Molly Allen, Elaine Koster, and Maryann Palumbo.

This book would not be possible without a successful practice. The success of this practice is a function of the motivation, intelligence, and kindness of its staff. They include Melissa, Helena, Gidion, and Lori. Chuck Cox is responsible for research for the book and projects within the practice.

Of special note, some special friends:
Gwen Barrett, Leonard Bernstein, Michael Cacoyannis, Jack Carney, Betty Comden, Steve Cuozzo, Edward Flanagan, Jan Goodwin, Barbara Gordon, Stuart Gorelick, Jane Hershey, Harriet Johnson, Kilpatrick family, Mrs. A. Lasker, Bernard Meltzer, Richard Mishaan, Irene Papas, Preston Phillips, Judy Price, Joe Saffon, Larry Schneider, Jack Schwartz, Marvin Scott, Vivian and Nat Serota, Ellen

Sills-Levy, Lise Spiegel, Linda Stasi, Carol Story, Geraldine Stutz, Phyllis and Alvin Trenk, Jeremy Wayne, Dan Weaver, Gordon Weaver, Anna Lee Wurlitzer, Jane and Steven Yohay

I have to thank my colleagues for their help on this book and in general:
Robert Atkins, MD, Ralph Berkeley, MD, Solomon Berson, MD, Joan Borysenko, PhD, William Cahan, MD, Janice Collins, LPN, Allan Cott, MD, Wilbur Gould, MD, Peter Herman, MD, Steven Herman, MD, Ruth Hersh, MED, Russell Jaffe, MD, Harold Karpman, MD, Martin Kurman, MD, Alberto Lopapa, MD, Alan Mandell, MD, Leslie-Jane Maynard, PhD, Mark Newman, MD, Linus Pauling, PhD, Theron Randolph, MD, Larry Rosenthal, DDS, Harvey Ross, MD, Cheryl Rush, Barry Saltzman, DO, Marina Saviotti, MD, Robert Schwartz, MD, Clarence Smith, MD, Hillel Tobias, MD, Kenneth Warren, MD

The core of the success has been the following patients who became friends:
Bella Abzug, Loretta Anderson, Roberta Balsam, Helen and Ralph Biernbaum, Leslie Brown, Arol Buntzman, Jay Burzon, Pat Cantwell, Karen and Anthony Cece, Certilman family, Nancy Chance, Cole family, Carolin Corbin, Ruth and Hans Clapper, Jim Dery, Joanne F. duPont, Marion Dystel, Suzy and Abba Eban, Irving Elias, Jack Elias, Alan Feinson, Louis Figueroa, Roberta Flack, Richard Flaxman, Alfred Flug, Mildred Fortinberry, Dot Fox, Ed Frankel, Friedman family, Vera and Nathan Garson, Ben Gazzara, Susan and Jonathan Giesberg, John Gilboy, Bernard Gittelson, Louis Goldberg, S. Howard Goldman, Arlene Goodman, Geoffrey Gordon, George Hamilton, Ellen Haynes, Jerry Herman, Craig Hollander, Emil Horowitz, Jane Pickens Hoving, Stewart Hutchinson, Marge Isselbacher, Joan Jablow-Frauenglass, Joan Katz, Kluger fam-

ily, Phyllis and Stanley Kreitman, Gary Lederman, Muriel Lederman, Reggie Leitman, Levien family, Beulah Levine, Flora Lewis, Rita and Howard Liebman, Carolyn Mann, Fran McCullough, Rochelle Melamed, Rhoda and Herbert Ment, Helen Meredith, Anne Meyer, Jane Wilkens Michael, Harvey Miller, Lucinda Mullin, Dario Negrini, Giulio Negrini, Helen Orens, Michael O'Shea, Estelle Ostrove, Phyllis Ottavano, David Pogrebin, Marcos Ponce, Frances Platzer, Dotson Rader, Joan Rosen, Walter Rosen, Billy Rudin, Anna Rugnetta, Lori Russo, Saccone family, Dorothy Sacks, Janet Sartin, Rita Schneider, Herb Schneiderman, Sendak family, Susan Shields, Estelle Silverstein, Gil Tunick, Renee Taylor, Ken Wagner, Paul Wattenberg, Ann Weiss, Rhoda Weissman, Emily Wilkens, Renee and Walter Wood

But most of all, I want to thank my parents, who with hard work, love, and support have given me the opportunity to practice medicine.

Contents

SECTION I

Get Ready for Immune Power

CHAPTER ONE

The Immune Power Diet Commitment

CONGRATULATIONS! Why? Because you have decided to become a healthier, happier, more vital person. You've taken the first step simply by beginning this book.

WHAT IS THE IMMUNE POWER DIET?

Here's what it is *not*. It is not a weight reduction plan, but you will quickly lose your unhealthy, unsightly excess pounds. It is not a fitness regime, but you will become stronger and more energetic. It is not a crash program, but you will experience renewed vitality in just a few weeks.

The Immune Power Diet is unique. *It is the first truly scientific nutritional plan designed to strengthen and revitalize your body's immune system.*

YOU ALREADY HAVE WHAT IT TAKES

The incredibly complex action, reaction, and interaction of trillions of cells in our bodies is called the immune system. It controls our ability to fight off disease and affects our levels of energy and creativity, even our moods and emotions. New breakthrough research shows that the immune system even affects our weight!

A new science has been born. Whether it is called preventive immunology, nutritional immunology, or immuno-modulation therapy, it is concerned with improving health by strengthening the body's own health-keeper, the immune system.

I've said that the immune system controls you, but this new science is proving—with discoveries reported at a breathtaking pace—that *you can affect your immune system by what you eat and what you DON'T eat. That's what my Immune Power Diet is all about.*

MOTHER KNEW BEST

Remember when your mother told you you had to eat right to stay strong and healthy? She said, "You'll weaken your constitution with all that junk! You'll get fat and lazy and dumb! You'll lower your resistance and you'll get sick!"

She was talking about *immunology*. Research biology has given us the tools to understand what your mother knew instinctively. We can now count immune cells with tests of exquisite sensitivity, measure blood chemicals to the millionth of a gram, quantify the biochemical reaction of our cells to our diet and even to aspects of our life-style.

I could not have written this book five, even three years ago, so new are these discoveries. I have used these dispatches from the frontiers of medicine and microbiology in my work with my patients to design and test a nutritional plan which can revitalize your immune system. The Immune Power Diet is based on cooperation, not competition, with your body's own extraordinary powers. It has been the prescription for health, weight loss, and super energy for over 3,000 of my patients. Do you want me to write a prescription for you?

ARE YOU READY TO MAKE THE IMMUNE POWER COMMITMENT?

- Are you ready to rid your body of toxins and chemicals that are sapping your vitality?
- Are you ready to stop having all those colds, bouts of flu, and other debilitating viral infections?
- Are you ready to lose unhealthy excess weight and become fit and strong?
- Are you ready to enjoy peak energy levels every day and enjoy restful, uninterrupted sleep?
- Are you ready to dump those vague aches and pains that drag you down?
- Are you ready to be more relaxed, responsive, and spontaneous with family, friends, and lovers?
- Are you ready to improve your powers of concentration and memory?
- Are you ready to start feeling positive about yourself?
- Are you ready to build for a long, healthy, active, successful life?

If your answers are YES, you have just made the Immune Power Diet commitment!

CHAPTER TWO

What's Ahead for You on the Immune Power Diet?

NOBODY STARTS a trip into unknown territory without a guide, so I'm going to give you a map right now that charts the rationale of the Immune Power Diet and outlines the methods you'll be using to fine-tune your immune system.

THE FIRST STEP— CORRECTING IMMUNE IMBALANCE

When your immune balance is upset, you open yourself to a whole range of illness, both acute and chronic. *The most frequent problems are caused by an immune hypersensitivity response to many of the foods we eat.*

I'll explain immune hypersensitivity fully in a later chapter, but for now, just remember that what you eat can damage your immune cells, creating or contributing to problems such as asthma, nausea, hives, anxiety, headaches, insomnia, heart palpitations, cramps, and swollen hands, feet or ankles.

Sometimes an immune imbalance makes our immune cells attack healthy parts of our bodies in what is called an *autoimmune response,* causing such common chronic problems as colitis, ulcers, dermatitis, and joint diseases.

When an inefficient immune system can't fight hard enough, we get recurrent diseases affecting the whole body, or diseases concentrated in specific organs such as the kidneys or lungs, or the reproductive system.

Everyone has a distinct set of immune reactions to various foods. Some food that we eat often—in fact, that we may crave—can do measurable, substantial damage to our immune cells. The range of immuno-toxic foods is large, and most importantly, differs from person to person. Your pattern of immuno-sensitivity to food is as unique as your fingerprints.

I have tested over a thousand of my patients for more than 150 of such hypersensitivities, and I have rarely discovered a patient without some significant immune damage created by some of the foods eaten regularly. It is virtually certain that *without being aware it is happening*, you are eating some foods that are damaging your immune system.

That's the bad news. *The good news is that I am going to show you how to identify these foods*. In Section II, I will take you step by step through the Introduction, Challenge, and Elimination Diet that will allow you to identify those damaging foods you were innocently introducing to your immune system. This is the same diet I prescribe for my patients, checking the results with sophisticated laboratory tests.

THE SECOND STEP— THE IMMUNE TUNE-UP

One of the most exciting breakthroughs in modern immunologic research is the growing evidence that your immune system holds the key to your weight as well as to your overall health.

The immune-fat connection is not so surprising, because we have long known that excess fat has damaging and even deadly effects throughout the body. It taxes the heart and lungs; blocks arteries, paving the way for a stroke or heart attack; weakens the liver, kidneys, and hormonal system; and may even promote disease such as diabetes and cancer. Recent studies have demonstrated that from 10 to 70 percent of cancer cases are related to obesity.

The immune system affects our weight in several ways: it regulates the manner in which we absorb, digest, and store food and how efficiently we can convert nutrients into energy. Fat is the body's natural energy reserve. The status of our immune system determines how much fat we burn for energy—or carry around in the form of excess weight. When your immune fat regulator needs a tune-up, you accumulate billions of extra fat cells. In Section II, I will show you how to break the immune-fat connection by following the Immune Power Diet plan. This is a simple regimen which allows you to eat a variety of delicious and healthful foods that encourage your immune system to turn you into a "lean machine" and keep you that way for life! (There are many alternatives on this diet so that you can adjust it to *your unique food hypersensitivities*.)

As a psychiatrist as well as a specialist in bariatrics (the science of weight control), I am well aware of the role fat plays in our mental as well as our physical health. In our culture, it is safe to say that to be fat is to be unhappy. Excess pounds all too often mean a tremendous load of excess psychological baggage to carry—feelings of guilt and shame at being out of control of your body, resentment and loneliness, and real or imagined sexual inadequacy.

But what do those attitudes have to do with our biological health? A great deal. There is increasing evidence that the link between our self-image and our biologic and immunologic well-being is very strong. According to research from such renowned medical centers as Stanford, Harvard, and UCLA, the immune system can be influenced by our mental attitudes. This means that *excess fat creates attitudes that can actually work to keep us unhealthy*. If you *believe* that you are fat and unhealthy, you will *stay* fat and unhealthy. *But*, you can break this vicious cycle by following the Immune Power Diet, eating the food your body needs to bring your immune system—and therefore your weight—into a healthful balance.

THE THIRD STEP—
REBUILDING YOUR IMMUNE SYSTEM

As you learn to identify the common foods that can damage your immune system, remove them from your diet, and lose excess weight, you will simultaneously be taking another important step toward a perfectly tuned, radically strengthened way of life. You will be *rebuilding* your immune defenses. This is accomplished through a carefully balanced plan of supplementation: vitamins, minerals, and amino acids, especially designed to fit your individual diet plan, life-style, sex, age, level of stress and immune-risk factors.

I have developed a simple system *that allows you to evaluate your immune status at any time*. You will use a checklist which I call the IQ test—not for intelligence but for your *Immune Quotient*.

As your IQ goes up, your supplementation goes down. But if you find yourself in a situation that threatens your immune system, you can supplement your IQ with special plans to rebuild your immunities. These special plans were devised to help you through rough times such as unusual stress or even grief, as well as to help with such common problems as pre-menstrual syndrome, or occasional over-indulgence in alcohol. I will even give you my personal formula for Nature's own appetite suppressant!

SAFETY FIRST

Many of the ideas in this book are highly controversial, because so much of the data derives from state-of-the-art research in immunology.

A growing number of medical educators and researchers believe that these new discoveries will profoundly influence future medical education and practice. But tomorrow's knowledge does you no good today. The Immune Power Diet puts the latest research findings to work for you *now* so that you can control your weight, boost your resistance to disease, and achieve superb health and vitality.

Still, with so much controversy, how can you know that the diet is safe? Easily. The Immune Power Diet is based on sound biological truths, entirely consistent with all the accepted principles of immunology. With the most rigorous science, the Immune Power Diet synthesizes what we now know about the interaction of food and immune cell function. As a practicing physician, I challenge anyone to find any aspect of this plan inconsistent with our understanding of immune health.

Yet, I am the first to admit that we don't know enough about this most exciting area of medicine. We are just beginning to learn how to recruit our body's own system to fight for better health. This book represents a first step on the road to understanding. Even I don't know *exactly* why the Immune Power Diet works so amazingly well.

When you compare the highly traumatic regimens commanded by most weight-loss manuals to the balanced harmony that is the basis of the Immune Power Diet, you will see why I don't want you to think of this as a diet book. Instead of a nutritional assault, the Immune Power Diet concentrates on rebuilding your natural systems. Following an eating plan which allows you to detoxify your body in combination with an individualized regimen of vitamins, minerals, and amino acids, based on your own immune status, the Immune Power Diet balances the system designed by the greatest biologist of them all.

Because it is a safe, harmonious approach, the Imune Power Diet is non-invasive and non-traumatic. *There is virtually no risk if you follow this program carefully.* As I've examined earlier, my nutritional plan cooperates, not competes, with medical treatments.

When a program shows such spectacular results with virtually no risk, it seems to me that as a physician, I have the responsibility to bring this proven program to the greatest number of people I can reach.

So what is this if not a diet book? It's an invitation to join a conspiracy, made up of you, your resolve, my knowledge and experience, and your natural health-keeper, the immune system. Its goal: to make you feel and look better than you ever imagined you could. If you're ready to conspire—to do yourself a favor and get healthy—let's begin.

CHAPTER THREE

Thirty-seven Tons Smart

SINCE I am asking you to make some big changes in your life, it's only fair to tell you something about the changes in my life that made me write this book. I once weighed *420 pounds*, so I know what it is like to live in a body that is grossly, inexcusably, overwhelmingly fat. Moreover, I know what it is to suffer from the myriad health problems—from headaches to ulcers to depression to joint problems—that come with being so fat.

I now weigh 208 pounds. That means I *know* what it feels like to steer oneself consciously, carefully, and successfully from ill-health to health and slimness.

LIVING ON THE FAT CYCLE

As the only son of parents who ran a Brooklyn candy store, I grew up in the care of a strict grandmother, isolated from friends my age. Lonely, and tempted by an endless supply of fattening foods, I soon learned the pattern that many of us learn as children: how to eat your way out of unhappiness.

I continued that destructive pattern through adolescence until, by age nineteen, I weighed an unbelievable 420 pounds. Even at 6'6½", there was no way I could "wear" all those extra pounds.

When the time came to start medical school, I was

worried. Even though I was a *summa cum laude* college graduate, the youngest member of my class at Tufts' medical school, and well on my way to becoming a physician, I knew my physical condition was sapping my strength and sabotaging my education and future career. It was turning my social and sexual relationships into a cruel joke.

There I was, looking more like a barn door than a young man of nineteen, huffing and wheezing as I struggled to cart my vast bulk around. I was getting little sleep and less exercise. My main physical activity consisted of opening the refrigerator to wolf down bulging fistfuls of junk food: cake, candy, chips—anything and everything to fill the cavernous void of my stomach.

With medical school's almost inhuman demands looming ahead, I knew something had to change, so I took matters into my own hands. As millions had before me, I made up my mind to get thin and get healthy. And, as millions had before me, I got into trouble.

The summer before medical school, I virtually stopped eating. Putting myself on a 300-calorie-a-day regime, I managed to drop forty pounds in five weeks.

I also nearly killed myself. After a few days, I could barely drag myself through the day. I felt my mind going fuzzy. It became hard, then impossible, to concentrate. I was swept by waves of nausea frequently through the day. My muscles grew so weak that I nearly fell when I stood up, and although I was more and more tired, I couldn't sleep.

In this state, I moved to Boston to enroll in medical school. I registered on a Tuesday morning, and found myself in a doctor's office that afternoon. She took one look at me, gasped, and gave it to me straight—my body was in a state of possibly lethal starvation. She rattled off the clinical signs: lethargy, confusion, pallor, faintness, poor muscle tone.

"Frankly," she said, "you are in no shape to start a

medical education. You've got a tough course ahead of you.'' She looked me right in the eye, ''If you ever want to heal anybody, you've got to start by taking care of your own health.'' I left her office with a diet she prescribed.

It was a traditional diet, counting calories, watching carbohydrates, balancing foods. And I *did* lose weight, but very slowly. I soon got over the signs of starvation but, as months went by, I wasn't getting any healthier. In fact, my health took a turn for the worse—much worse.

SICKER AND SICKER

First came terrible stomach pains. I figured they were due to the stresses of medical school, so I ignored them. They grew more frequent and painful until, one day, I was rushed to the emergency room. I had arrived, I later learned, bleeding profusely from my stomach. It took six pints of blood to stop the life-threatening hemorrhage. The diagnosis: a duodenal ulcer.

My recovery was agonizing. I was in the intensive care ward where the doctors had put me on potent stomach drugs. These antacids, I knew from my training, could cause kidney disease. At the same time, they were giving me another drug, a very common ulcer medicine, which I knew could make me impotent. Once back in school, I found myself distracted from my school work by the constant pain in my stomach.

Then came a new set of troubles. Suddenly, I started falling into bleak, despairing moods, periods where I had no energy and the world seemed awful. These alternated with phases of manic over-excitement, and I soon found myself on a roller coaster of depression and elation. Worse, I was having tremendous difficulty concentrating on my work. My mind was as fuzzy as it had been when I was starving myself.

Then came the headaches. In my second year at Tufts, I began having a series of excruciating migraines. They came on without warning, in the middle of lecture or in the lab, so severe that I had to stop whatever I was doing and lie down. My doctors tried every test but found nothing wrong, although my headaches became more and more frequent and debilitating.

Finally, I was so incapacitated with pain that the doctors suggested I undergo a myelogram, a risky and painful procedure in which dye is injected into the brain through the spinal cord. Terrified that my headaches might be caused by a brain disease or tumor, I submitted to the procedure.

While it proved negative—to my vast relief!—it had a devastating sequel. I couldn't lift my head without a crippling, searing, exploding pain, so intense that every time I stood up or turned my head I would become nauseated.

Now I was worse off than ever before. While trying to study, I learned that whenever I lifted my head even a few inches, the pain made the words swim on the paper, and I couldn't write. I will never forget the awful ordeal of my finals that year. I received special permission to take them lying on the floor, so that I could read and finish the questions without losing consciousness.

Never had I felt so frustrated. I worked, studied, and lived at a center of medical knowledge, in a hive of Nobel prize-winning physicians and medical scientists. But my many doctors disagreed over what was wrong with me, and the various treatments only made me sicker. I felt that if I continued, I would have to drop out of school, or that I might end up insane, or dead.

Now, for the second time, I decided to take matters into my own hands. The doctors clearly didn't know what to do, so I set out to design my own health plan.

DISCOVERING THE IMMUNE CONNECTION

First, I set out to learn everything I possibly could about the physiological, biochemical, immunological, and psychological aspects of nutrition and weight loss. In addition to attending medical school, I enrolled in the Harvard School of Public Health.

The more I studied, the more excited I became. Every single finding, every study and research report, could be related exactly to the very problems that had made my life such agony. Mood and emotions, obesity, stomach and nerve problems, headaches . . . I began to see the *direct nutritional connections* that explained all of them.

Each question I asked led me to a series of fascinating answers. How, I wondered, does nutrition affect us in disease and health? I discovered work by Dr. Robert Good, one of the premier immunologists of the age, then Director of New York's Memorial Sloan-Kettering Cancer Center. Dr. Good showed that diets high in fat could speed up the shrinking of the thymus, a vital organ that processes our immune cells. What's more, such a diet also fostered tremendous imbalances in the immune system and brought on a number of destructive diseases. In short, I realized that *reducing fat in the diet actually meant we could forestall the ravages of many common diseases*.

From research done at the U.S. Army Medical Research Institute of Infectious Diseases I began to learn about the links between specific nutrients and the immune system. A lack of vitamin B_6 for example, creates a serious deficiency in the body's disease-fighting cells. Insufficient vitamin C was shown to impair the body's ability to keep itself well.

Dr. R. K. Chandra at MIT reported that minerals, zinc,

for example, are essential strengtheners of the body's health-keeping immune cells. I learned that vitamin E stimulates a range of defensive functions, increasing our ability to fight infection and cancer.

I became familiar with the research on what scientists call *free radicals*. It's a dramatic-sounding name, bringing to mind visions of escaped terrorists. Well, that's not so far wrong, for free radicals are highly unstable byproducts created as our cells use oxygen. Because they are so unstable, they react easily with many chemicals inside the cells, and these reactions can cause tremendous damage to the delicate cellular control mechanisms. When those mechanisms are damaged, the cell may malfunction or die. Biologists tell us that this cumulative cell damage is the cause of many of the common degenerative diseases: arthritis, hardening of the arteries, heart and kidney ailments.

Reading the research, I learned that vitamins like C, E, and A seem to act to "sponge up" free radicals, scooping them up before they can commit cellular sabotage. This is one reason why such vitamins seem to strengthen our immune system and help prevent many common diseases.

BEING MY OWN MOUSE

Of course, everything that I was learning came straight from the world's most advanced research laboratories. Many of these discoveries, especially in immunology, have since been clinically proven, but at the time, it was all so new that most of our knowledge was still in the "white mice" laboratory phase. Nobody really knew how—or if—these findings actually worked in people.

So, I had no choice but to become my own mouse. I tried varying specific elements of my diet, observing what happened. I experimented with foods, vitamins, minerals, protein, carbohydrates, fiber, and amino acids—in short, every part of the human diet. I kept meticulous track of the results.

I saw that I felt better and was sick less when I took a steady regimen of vitamins C, A, and E. My mood and energy stabilized when I ate specific kinds of proteins, while it went into a tailspin when I ate large amounts of sugars or carbohydrates. My nerves became calm and I slept better when I took B Complex vitamins and certain amino acids. I noticed that I felt irritable and tired when I ate wheat and dairy products, and that by avoiding them, my feelings of well-being and my energy increased.

BACK TO BASICS, BACK TO HEALTH

I soon realized that I was far better off than when I was undergoing traditional medical treatments. All those years of agonizing tests, of invasive, traumatic procedures and highly toxic medications had left me sick, weak, still obese, and exhausted. Now, following my own hybrid system, I was losing more weight, and feeling better, than I ever had.

When I finished medical school, I weighed a comfortable 210 pounds. On my tall frame, that meant I looked trim, well-proportioned, and athletic. I had lost over 200 pounds—the weight of two average women! But for all I'd lost, I'd gained something even more vital: having seen exactly half of me melt away, and feeling healthier and more energetic than I ever had on a weight-loss plan of my own design, *I knew it could be done*.

Finishing with a specialty in psychiatry, I continued my research into bariatrics, the science of weight control. As a student at Harvard, I plunged even deeper into all areas of nutrition and the psychology of weight control.

I knew from my own experience that weight loss depends on a delicate balance of diet, exercise, nutrition, and attitude. I started working on the idea of manipulating appetite with natural vitamins and amino acids instead of dangerous drugs like amphetamines.

MORE IMMUNE CLUES

I studied the links between the amino acids in our diet and our immune system. At MIT, researchers were showing that the body uses amino acids (the basic chemical building blocks that make up the proteins we eat) to help build the cells that fight infections. Among those amino acids, tryptophan, phenylalanine, and valine appear particularly crucial to the production of strong antibodies which are the core of the body's defense against viruses and bacteria. Other amino acids help build other blood cells that defend us against deadly viruses, fungi, and bacteria, and help to fight cancer.

I familiarized myself with research done at the Karolinska Institute in Sweden, home of the Nobel Prize in medicine. There, doctors found that obese people are more susceptible to a wide range of serious bacterial infections. This coincided with the work of Dr. Newberne at MIT, who found that the more fat a body has, the greater the likelihood of serious infections. His work also concurs with other studies that have linked obesity to cancer.

Feeling that my experience—personal, medical, and psychiatric—provided a unique blend of credentials to help others lose weight, I incorporated many of these findings into my first book.

WHY A NEW DIET?

When I wrote that first book, it represented years of research and clinical experience. However, new research reports flowing in from my colleagues at major medical centers around the world documented far more about the subtle interplay of nutrition, health, and weight loss than had been known when I wrote that book. Each day, it seemed, I learned of yet another state-of-the-art discovery, some sweeping new breakthrough. Provocative new findings in immunology, preventive medicine, and nutrition were almost exploding out of the research laboratories! I realized my first book had not gone far enough. But that wasn't all. My Fifth Avenue practice had become deluged with patients, and those patients taught *me* a tremendous amount.

I began to realize that my patients fall into three types. The first are truly desperate. Many of them suffer from the same debilitating symptoms I had: declining energy and alertness, headaches, stomach and intestinal syndromes, lethargy and fatigue, skin disorders—all with no clear explanation. Often, they came to me because they simply didn't know where else to turn. I know from my experience how powerless and bitter many of these people feel as they watch their health slip away, never knowing why.

The second group of patients had come for a wholly different reason. For these people, it is no luxury to feel, act, and look their best—it is an absolute necessity. These are film and television celebrities, major power brokers from Wall Street, corporate heavy hitters who sit at the helms of empires like Paramount Pictures and Morgan Stanley. These are the world-renowned artists, musicians, intellectuals, professional athletes, and members of the ruling families of several continents.

These people know that their health is their most valuable capital for success: they must look and perform flawlessly at all times. Their minds must brim with energy, creativity, and inspiration to meet the challenges of the world's most demanding careers. They have come to me to tune their bodies to a perfect pitch of health and vitality.

I have a third group of patients, just regular people, who consult me because of a nagging feeling that they could be healthier and more energetic. They have no specific complaints, just the vague suspicion that they lack the get-up-and-go and fun in their lives that others enjoy.

Most of my patients share the same frustration. They have already tried a grueling round-robin of the ''best'' specialists, clinics, and therapies by the time they get to my waiting room. They are here because they have tried to get help elsewhere, but failed to find any.

ON THE TRAIL
OF AN IMMUNE MYSTERY

The more I thought about it, the more I realized that these different groups of patients who, at first glance, seemed absolutely dissimilar had something in common. Two very peculiar things stood out.

First, in the course of routine blood tests, I found that many of my patients who wanted to lose weight also had severe imbalances in their immune system. Test samples drawn from what seemed to be healthy arms showed blood profiles that were in immunological shambles. Equally intriguing, not all of my patients responded the same way to treatment. Patients often seemed to get better up to a point, but then get stuck. I was treating a puzzling range of complaints: unexplained ailments, skin rashes and lesions, and, particularly, profound psychological problems, including depression, anxiety, and lethargy. I found that patients' symptoms would lessen or disappear, but I didn't see the clear improvement in overall health that I expected.

Others lost weight perfectly well, but that was as far as I went. Although they were pleased with their weight loss, I had the feeling they were stopping at some vague halfway point—that something was blocking them from getting robustly healthy.

And there were a few, too, who simply couldn't lose much weight at all, in spite of the fact that I was using every traditional tool and technique known to bariatric medicine. I worked desperately to find the clues to solve this medical mystery.

SHARON'S THUMB

What finally cracked the case was Sharon's thumb. When Sharon first came to my office, she was on the verge of tears. I listened as she poured out her story. She had worked for twenty years building her career as one of New York's best designers of custom furs. She worked with her hands constantly doing precise hand stitching, stacking coats on racks, and lifting heavy pelts. Recently, she had been troubled by pain and stiffness in her hands, particularly in her right thumb. At first, it had been just inconvenient, she explained, and she had tried, on her physician's orders, taking aspirin and anti-inflammatory drugs. But they did little good, and the pain grew worse. On many days, her pain was so severe that she couldn't work. She was desperate.

"Furs are all I know, doctor. It's my career, my life. I don't know what I could do if I had to give it up."

She was also concerned about her weight, and rightly so. Her small frame carried at least forty excess pounds, which made her seem much older than her years. Despair was in her voice as she described the many diets, on which she had tried—and failed—to lose weight. As we talked, I began to suspect that her severe weight problem was linked to the trouble she was having with her hands. I ordered a test to see if she had any hidden food allergies.

Food allergies are a very widespread and very unrecognized problem. Recent research has just begun to show us that each of us has allergies to certain foods. When we eat these foods they react with the white cells in our blood that are a part of the immune system, damaging or killing hundreds of thousands of these vital protectors. Our food allergies are as varied as the range of foods we eat, but each person's specific sensitivities are unique. In fact, they are so individual that they make up a unique biochemical "fingerprint." Until recently, we didn't have the sophisticated laboratory tests to see this damage actually occur, but thanks to technological advances, we now can.

The test I gave Sharon exposes a small blood sample to hundreds of food extracts. By watching how the patient's immune cells react to different foods, we can test hundreds of foods quickly and efficiently for their allergy potential.

Her tests showed that many of the foods she ate every day—corn, yeast, certain vegetables, and fish—were actually killing her white blood cells, causing not only her chronic symptoms but her weight problem. I explained that by removing these toxic foods from her diet, there was a chance her symptoms would stop.

Three weeks later, I picked up the phone to hear an ecstatic Sharon on the line, "This is unbelievable! The pain in my hand has completely disappeared. I'm back working with no problem at all!" When I saw her two months later, she had lost a total of thirty-nine pounds, the same pounds she had worked to lose in vain for years. Looking at this slim, energetic woman, I hardly recognized the person who had been on the verge of tears in my office. "I still can't believe it. Here I was, all those years, keeping myself fat and sick, just by eating wrong!"

THE BIRTH OF
THE IMMUNE POWER DIET

It was then that I realized just how promising this new principle was, not just for Sharon, but for everyone. I took what I had learned from Sharon and applied these principles to some of my other patients, focusing their treatment not simply on weight loss but on rebuilding damaged immune systems.

I scrutinized the diet, life-style, and stress level of all my patients because each of these affect immune function. I devised special diets to remove a patient's individual toxic foods. Then, I used all of nature's nutritional building blocks—vitamins, amino acids, and minerals—to rebuild their damaged immune systems.

The more I refined treatment based on individual immune responses, the broader improvements I saw in *every* area of my patients' health. No matter why they had first consulted me, they became more alert, vital, happier, and less prone to infection. *And,* they lost weight. Truly, *healthy immune cells mean a healthy person.*

BREAKING THE FAT CYCLE

I have treated more than 3,000 patients since making this discovery, and I know that the Immune Power Diet works. Those who follow this nutrition plan become healthier, have a better mental state, and get thin. And they don't just get thin—they *stay* thin. Initial weight loss is important, but keeping that weight off is critical.

This treatment has proven the modality of choice for steady long-term maintenance. This is because the Immune Power Diet is specifically designed to balance the body's immune system, creating what biologists call *homeostasis*—"self-regulation."

Nutritional peaks and valleys are smoothed out, food cravings and the need to binge uncontrollably are eliminated.

THE BOTTOM LINE

I've tried to wear four hats here. I've personally felt the agony and frustration of spending half of my life grossly fat and profoundly unhealthy. Knowing my own misery during that period, I have a personal stake in making sure that my patients won't have to waste valuable years feeling unhealthy and unloved.

As a physician, rigorously trained at Tufts and Harvard, I know my nutrition plan must incorporate only proven, safe medical principles.

The Hippocratic Oath, which each graduating physician must take, reminds us: "Above all else, do no harm." That became my guiding principle. Both my sense of medical ethics and my professional reputation among my research colleagues demands that nothing in this plan ever could, in any way, endanger patients.

As a psychiatrist, I know that no matter how biologically sound a nutrition program is, it will only work if it takes into account all that we encompass: our needs and fears, family and peer support, individual life-style, and commitment to making real behavior changes. These all must be orchestrated for any true growth to take place, so I have built in the principles of psychological health which help people to make positive changes in their lives.

But most important, as one who makes his living every day by helping people get healthy and lose weight, I knew this plan had to *work for everyone*.

This brings me to a statistic I'm very proud of: in the recent years that I have used the Immune Power Diet, I have helped over 3,000 of my patients lose a total of more than *74,000* pounds of extra weight. *Seventy-four thousand pounds*. That's *37 tons* of fat. Enough fat to fill a dozen dumptrucks. Every one of those pounds—mine and my patients'—has taught me a lesson about effective, safe, and health-promoting weight control.

This book is based on my scientific study and research over the last decade, but I owe its inspiration to something much more personal: to those 37 tons of lessons from all those different patients.

CHAPTER FOUR

Invincible You: A Short Course in Immune Appreciation

IT SHOULD BE clear by now that your immune system is the key to better health, to more energy and enjoyment, and to safe, permanent, weight control. But what exactly *is* your immune system, anyway? Obviously, to bring this system into perfect tone—and yourself into perfect health—you must understand something of what it is and how it works. That's what this chapter is about. I'm going to show you what goes on in the magnificent network of cells and chemicals that make up your immune system. With this knowledge you can get the most out of the Immune Power Diet, and make your health and vitality flourish as you lose weight. I promise, after reading about your immune system, you'll never see your body quite the same way again.

IMMUNOLOGY 101

You probably already know that the immune system is the body's defender: it identifies, tracks down, and destroys biological troublemakers before they can damage the body. Those troublemakers may be, for example, bacteria from a cut or splinter, a measles germ, a cold bug, a deadly rare fungus, or even a cancer cell.

These "invaders" try to take over our tissues and feed off our body's nutrients. If they succeed, we become sick or, sometimes, even die. It's your immune system's job to destroy these invaders before they destroy you.

MEET YOUR FOUR VITAL IMMUNE FRIENDS

The immune system is tremendously complex, but there are really only four key parts of it that you need to understand in order to put the principles of the Immune Power Diet to work for you. They are: the thymus, the T cells (a special kind of white cells, or *lymphocytes*), antibodies, and macrophages ("scavenger cells"). Rather than give you a biology lesson, I'll introduce this cast of characters by showing you just what they do inside you.

Say you picked up a flu virus last week. Perhaps it entered your body through a cut, from a drinking glass, or just from the air you breathe. Of course, you never felt it at all, but the virus stealthily made its way into your bloodstream, constantly replicating. These viruses have one goal: to take over your cells. Inside your body's warm corridors, they will try to enter crucial cells and disrupt their normal work. Eventually, left unchecked, these viruses would damage so many cells that you would weaken, or worse, become seriously ill.

But this marauding flu virus didn't count on your immune system. As it multiplies in your bloodstream, it is met by a certain kind of white blood cell, the lymphocytes. Lymphocytes are the crucial foot soldiers in the immune battle that keep you alive. Remember these cells because you'll be hearing a lot more about them in this book, because keeping *them* healthy is the key to keeping *you* healthy. Later on, you'll see how what you eat can dramatically help or hurt your vital lymphocyte protectors.

IMMUNE FIGHTERS

Lymphocytes teem in numbers that tax the imagination. Thousands of them could fit in the period at the end of this sentence. Your body holds about a trillion—that's 1,000,000,000,000—of them, or about 3,000 in every drop of blood. Since you began this very sentence, over 800,000 of them have been created and destroyed.

Some of these lymphocytes pass through a small, walnut-sized organ at the base of your neck called the thymus. Here, special hormones turn lymphocytes into aggressive fighting cells, called T cells ("T" for thymus—immunology isn't so complicated after all). You'll be hearing more about the thymus, too, because what you eat directly affects how well this organ makes the T cells you need to keep healthy.

These immune cells have one terrific talent: they can distinguish friend from foe, what should be in our bodies from what shouldn't. They do not affect the body's healthy cells, yet they attack everything that is foreign to our bodies such as germs, transplants and grafts, even our own cells which have turned malignant.

IMMUNE RED ALERT!

Whenever an immune cell encounters a trespasser, it slots into it like a key into a lock, holds on tight, and sounds the alarm. That's what happens if a flu virus enters your body. As soon as your immune sentries raise the alarm, the troops swing into action.

First, T cells start reproducing in order to outnumber the virus. Each new T cell is programmed to fight this exact enemy. Some of these cells, the "natural killer" (NK) cells, surround the cells where the invading virus has hidden. NK cells attack your virus-contaminated cells, in a sense suffocating them. They release deadly chemicals that make the cells burst.

Now chemical messengers are sent to summon aid for your body's first line of defense. As these chemicals concentrate at the site, the area begins to redden, swell, and get tender. These are the signs of an infection. The same reaction creates the muscular and joint aches you feel when you are sick. Some of the chemicals released signal the brain to raise the body's temperature to make the immune cells work faster—and so you run a fever.

Now you feel the familiar "swollen glands." These really aren't glands at all, but collection points along the network of tubes that transport the immune cells pouring forth to fight the invader. The tube system is called the *lymph system,* and the collection points are *lymph nodes.* When they get large and tender, that means battalions of immune cells are mustering for battle. Rather than a sign for alarm, such an inflammation shows that the body is doing its normal job, and that a ferocious battle is raging within.

By now, the invaders are probably wondering how they ever got into this mess as they are outnumbered by attacking T cells and surrounded by blood chemicals helping those cells. What else could go wrong?

I'm glad you asked. Because right about now your immune troops bring on a new weapon: the *antibodies.* Antibodies are tuned like guided missiles to hone in on the invader, and thousands of them pour into the bloodstream every second. They zoom in, surround the virus and hold on for dear life. (You'll be hearing more about antibodies, too, because if your body lacks certain nutrients, it won't do a very good job of making the antibody "missiles" you need.)

Enter the last fighter in the immune battle, the *macrophages,* another kind of white blood cell. Their name means, literally, "big eater," and that's exactly what they do. Whenever they see something covered with antibody— that is, an invader—they lumber up and "eat" it.

With so many immune defenders at work, the virus doesn't have a chance. It is ganged up on by T cells, antibodies, macrophages, and all the blood chemicals that the immune system recruits. With all this tumult going on inside you, it's no wonder you feel so tired when you get the flu!

SCORE—YOU: 1, INVADER: 0

When the smoke clears, the invaders have been destroyed. Now your immune troops reduce, your glands shrink, the aches, pains, and fever disappear. The sentries drift back to routine patrol. And you get out of bed and go back to work, taking for granted your good health, not knowing what a valiant battle your immune soldiers have fought on your behalf.

These immune battles rage every second of every day, without stop. Because our bodies contain many trillions of microorganisms, our immune system is engaged in constant battle for as long as we live.

Sometimes the threat isn't from outside invaders; sometimes our own cells turn pre-cancerous. No matter—your immune cells treat these traitors the same way. The eminent Dr. Lewis Thomas, former Director of Memorial

Sloan-Kettering Cancer Center in New York, helped pioneer our understanding of this immune surveillance. His work helped show how the immune cells keep constant patrol to locate and destroy cells that have mutated—that is, changed from their normal form. If the immune system is impaired, these cells can turn into cancer.

THE CRUCIAL IMMUNO-NUTRITION LINK

So, now you see why these four parts of the immune system are the key to your overall health. But what does nutrition have to do with all of this? That's easy; what you eat can either strengthen or weaken your immune system.

It is no surprise that the immuno-nutrition link is crucial. Your body creates 200,000 new immune cells every second of your life and thousands of antibody molecules also have to be made every second. This adds up to millions of cells that the body must rebuild daily.

It is absolutely essential that your body get the nutrients it needs to stay battle-ready at all times. What we eat provides the body with the vital elements to build those millions of immune cells. These are: amino acids, proteins, minerals, and vitamins.

Vitamins, for example, play a key role at every stage of the immune battle. The most recent research shows that a lack of vitamin A lowers the number of T cells—which means fewer immune soldiers to mount an attack. Without enough of the B vitamins—particularly B_6 and B_{12}—your cells can't make crucial germ-fighting antibodies, and that means one less arm of defense. Vitamin C has been shown in many studies to be crucial to macrophage activity—because without it, these crucial "cell-eaters" can't do a good job.

Minerals, too, profoundly affect different parts of the immune system. Zinc is perhaps the most vital immune mineral. Without enough zinc in our bodies, many of the lymph system tissues actually shrink, including the thymus where crucial T cells develop, and the lymph nodes where immune soldiers are stored. The concentration of zinc in our cells also affects how energetically the macrophages attack invaders, and studies have shown that low zinc likewise reduces the numbers of T cells. Other minerals are also important. Insufficient selenium reduces antibodies in test animals, and too much copper, cadmium, or lead can actually weaken T cells, so they don't fight invaders efficiently.

Amino acids are also crucial. Tryptophan, phenylalanine, lysine, and methionine are necessary to the production of antibody. And because amino acids are the building blocks for all of the body's cells, they clearly affect how many T cells we will have available to fight off invading germs and cancer.

There are over fifty such crucial immune nutrients, and they must be in precise balance for our immune defenses to work powerfully and efficiently.

THE MIND FACTOR

Fascinating findings now coming out of research centers show that we can actually affect our immune system when we have a concrete picture of how it works. This trailblazing new science is called *psychoneuroimmunology:* the study of how attitudes affect immune health. Dr. Carl Simonton and his wife Stephanie are the best known pioneers in this vanguard science. They find that the very act of specifically, concretely picturing what's happening in the immune system can sometimes actually make it perform better. The Simontons augment conventional cancer treatment with a technique called "guided imagery." At the Simonton clinic in Ft. Worth, patients are taught how to imagine very concrete images of their immune system fighting cancer, and encouraged to visualize that action as graphically as possible. Some patients envision knights on white horses, others see tanks and fighter planes —the details don't matter, so long as they have a clear picture.

In a significant number of cases, the results have been dramatic. Tumors shrink, symptoms disappear, and the patients' mental states improve dramatically. Nobody knows exactly how these mental images boost the immune system, but several researchers have consistently reported that the technique can improve both physical and psychological health.

THE HIDDEN IMMUNE FACTOR

There is one final way in which the foods you eat can profoundly help or hurt your immune protectors. Certain foods we all eat—foods that seem nourishing and healthy—can actually cause thousands of our vital lymphocytes to explode. We can clearly record and measure these reactions. If you could look in my laboratory microscope, you would see the vital lymphocyte cells—the core of our immune defense—swell and self-destruct when exposed to certain food toxins.

Because this work is so new (much of it is being refined as this book goes to press) there's still much to learn. But we know that these reactions cause a whole range of physical and psychological problems. They can also touch off a chronic eating binge reaction, we actually crave the very foods that do the most damage to our cells. This, in turn, sets off a physiological chain reaction that makes us gain weight.

THE MORAL OF THE STORY: EAT FOR YOUR CELLS

What we eat is the single largest area in which we can affect our immune system. Now that you have seen the four key components of your immune well-being, you understand that you can, and must, eat to help your immune power function at its peak. Your cells can help keep you healthy, vital, alert and energetic, feeling and looking young . . . *if* you eat to give them what they need.

CHAPTER FIVE

Fats, Fads, and Immune Health

Now IS the time to take a hard look at a tender subject: your waistline. And, for that matter, your thighs, hips, tummy, arms, ankles—any place your body keeps its unsightly, and unhealthy, fat bank accounts.

WHERE DO YOU HAVE YOUR FAT BANK ACCOUNTS?

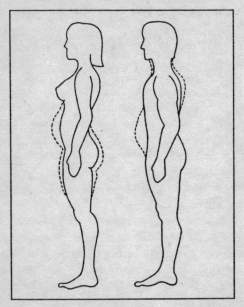

Fat storage depends on many factors, including your sex, and men and women store fat differently. Take a look at where you have your own fat bank account.

TAKE THE PINCH TEST

You can get a rough-and-ready measure of your "immune tune" by using my *pinch test*. Using your thumb and forefinger, take a pinch of your waistline. If you feel more than ½-inch of extra fat, you know your body's weight control system has banked too much energy in your fat reserves. The needless energy reserves created by an out-of-tune immune system leave you, quite literally, sitting on your fat assets.

IMMUNO-FITNESS AND FAT

The fat you can pinch is just the tip of the iceberg. Within your body, fat cells, unleash a destructive tug-of-war between you and your immune system. This fat-immune cycle works simply: the fatter you are, the worse shape your immune system is in, and the more you get sick. If you are overweight, you are more vulnerable to colds, flu, serious infections, viral diseases, heart disease, diabetes, and cancer.

And, the worse your "immune tune," the easier it will be to get fat and stay that way. That means *each extra pound you carry actually makes it harder to lose weight and, conversely, easier to gain it*. As you can imagine, this creates a terrible, self-perpetuating cycle in which poor health and excess weight contribute to each other.

OVERWEIGHT   IMMUNE DAMAGE

- Eating disorders
- Medical problems
- Low energy and stamina

- Mood swings
- Frequent illness
- Weakness

- Health problems
- Faster aging

This vicious cycle is like being stuck on a merry-go-round you can't escape. But it's anything but "merry." Diane, one of my patients, came up with the perfect name for this cycle: the Fat Dreary-Go-Round.

Diane knew the "dreary-go-round" only too well. For the last fifteen years, her excess weight had fluctuated between 35 and 45 pounds. Because she had been quite slim and vivacious as a younger woman, she was well aware of the toll her fat was levying on her energy, her spirit and sense of self, and even her relationship with her husband.

Over the years, Diane had tried every possible plan to shed the pounds that were making her life so grim. She tried fasting and eating only fruits. She tried an all-protein diet, and made herself sick on a protein-sparing diet; she had run the gamut of the Scarsdale, high-protein, and macrobiotic diets.

But no matter what she tried, nothing worked. She saw herself growing increasingly lethargic, depressed, and troubled by worsening arthritis in her hands. Worst of all, she confided, her spreading bulk had completely cooled her husband's sexual interest. At every level of her life, Diane knew only too well the fat cycle "dreary-go-round."

On her second visit to my office, Diane decided to make a commitment to the Immune Power Diet way to lose weight.

In fourteen weeks, Diane lost the thirty-five pounds that she had struggled unsuccessfully to lose for so many years. These were the pounds that had been keeping her from doing what she really wanted to do most in the world: say good-bye to her "dreary-go-round."

TAKE YOURSELF OFF THE DREARY-GO-ROUND

By power-tuning your immune system, you can reverse the insidious immune-fat cycle. You can stop your immune fighters from working against you, and enlist them on your side to lose weight, and gain better health and greater energy.

In order to break the vicious immune-fat cycle, you must understand how this catastrophic cycle gets started. The field of *lipid immunology*—the science of fat and immune health—is so revolutionary that it is still largely uncharted.

But one thing is clear: millions of people out there continue doggedly to count calories, yet cannot lose weight.

Recent studies sponsored by the National Science Foundation show that calories simply are not the key to weight loss that we once believed.

The common pattern is well-known to every one who has ever tried to lose weight: an impressive initial weight loss followed by a long plateau of little or no loss. The reason for this is clear: without proper understanding of the key immune role in weight loss, you can't hope to break the insidious cycle that keeps you fat.

There's no question that the immune-fat cycle is real, and that it works. I have seen well over three thousand patients like Diane who have had extraordinary results once they recruited their immune systems to help them lose weight. Those patients have shown for certain that there's a strong link between a strong immune system and a slim waistline.

The evidence that excess fat directly, and severely, weakens your immune system is alarming and overwhelming. It means that:

- Fat people get sick more.
- Fat people suffer more debilitating headaches, joint pain, stomach upset, and skin problems.
- Fat people are more prone to depression, mood changes, fatigue, and lethargy.
- Fat people age faster and are more vulnerable to chronic debilitating diseases like diabetes, cancer, and heart disease.
- Fat people have less energy, stamina, and resilience.

In short, fat people become less healthy and stay less healthy because their immune system is less healthy.

FATS AND FADS

Should we then go to any extreme to rid ourselves of excess weight as quickly as possible? That's the rationale behind many of the wild fad diets which have become popular over the years. But unfortunately, it's not as simple as that. This kind of crisis reasoning can lead to all manner of medically unwise, risk-laden diets. The "fat crisis" diets have one thing in common: they disrupt the body's metabolic cycle. They are designed to throw the body into a sudden state of shock in order to achieve weight loss.

But your extra inches didn't come on overnight, and they won't disappear that way either. You can't hope to get rid of fat, and keep it off, unless you remove the underlying cause of fat—the bad equilibrium that gave you all that extra baggage to begin with.

As I write this, I have beside me a stack of scientific papers showing that dietary fads can lead to significant immune deficiency. Ironically, these weight-loss diets can disturb your immune system so much that they actually push you downward into the immune-fat spiral.

Phyllis was a perfect example of this. Soon after she had her first child in her late twenties, she started on a conscientious diet and exercise program to get her figure back. It worked well, and she regained almost the same slim profile she had enjoyed before. But when, at age thirty-four, she bore her second daughter, it didn't quite work that way.

Maybe it was having another small child to care for, or just being a few years older, but Phyllis just didn't bounce back the same way. Instead of firming up again as she had after her first child, she steadily lost control of her weight altogether. By the time her second baby was six months old, Phyllis had gained an extra twenty-two pounds. She felt chronically tired and short of breath, whether doing errands in town, or just going up and downstairs at home. Every week, she saw two more pounds registering on her bathroom scale.

Because she had always been a take-charge type, Phyllis decided to attack her weight head-on, and when a girlfriend recommended a popular diet, she brought it home, and read it that same night.

She plunged immediatly into the diet, paring her menu and her food portions down to the minimum the diet required. At first, the pounds slipped off, so she didn't worry as she began to notice her energy flagging even more than before. Now, instead of slowing down half-way through the day, she was tired and groggy when she woke up. She started having nagging headaches—nothing debilitating, but steady, constant throbbing. After ten days, or so, her fair skin looked dry and tired, and her hands had developed a slight shake that worsened as the day wore on. Although she was worried, she stayed with the diet, still desperate to lose weight.

Then, one Thursday afternoon as Phyllis was working in her office, she stood up to retrieve a file, and was overcome by dizziness. "I felt like a wave at the beach had hit me," she remembered. As she grabbed the edge of her desk to steady herself, nausea hit her. "That was when I really got scared for the first time. I've never felt so weak." She was in my office the next day.

One look at her reminded me of how I must have looked to my own doctor long ago. Her eyes were sunken, she was pale and agitated, and her skin hung loosely. This was a woman who had malnourished herself to the edge of very serious trouble, because she was totally determined to lose weight.

Phyllis left my office that day with an entirely new perspective: from now on, she would eat to help her body lose weight—not fight against her natural nutritional needs. When I saw her four weeks later, she had lost fourteen pounds, and she continues to make steady progress, while enjoying renewed health and vitality.

That is the whole point of the Immune Power Diet. It uses a balanced program to lose weight safely, sanely, in a way that uses the body's own self-regulating mechanism. The Immune Power Diet uses many nutritional elements. But the two most important nutritional keys to help you get thin *now* are high fiber and complex carbohydrates.

FIBER: FILLING, NOT FATTENING

Fiber helps you lose weight in two main ways. First, it simply fills you up. Physiologically, bulky food means you will feel less hungry, and you will eat less of the high-calorie, high-sugar and fatty foods that put on pounds and damage your immune system.

Moreover, a high-fiber diet helps smooth out the peaks and valleys of protein and sugar digestion. That means less erratic eating patterns, more constant high energy, and a more stable, positive mood. High fiber also helps you to avoid wild binges on high-sugar foods, and by preventing these destructive food binges, you can break another link in the subtle immune-fat cycle.

All of the recipes in Section Two have been designed to include an excellent balance of fiber to strengthen your immune fighters, reduce food binges, and lower your weight.

COMPLEX CARBOHYDRATES: THE TIME-RELEASE WAY TO LOSE WEIGHT

The complex carbohydrate foods such as pasta, potatoes, and whole grains are a key part of this diet. Like sugars, these foods are high in energy, but unlike sugar, they break down slowly in our bodies. In effect, they work as time-release energy sources. Not long ago, foods like potatoes, rice, and pasta were definitely *verboten* in any weight-loss program, but today, we appreciate the role complex carbohydrates play in weight loss, fitness, and a healthy immune system.

Much of that new knowledge has come from the people

who must keep their health at a perfect pitch: professional athletes. Advanced sports medicine professionals have taught us how truly vital complex carbohydrates are to maintaining high energy, stamina, and the overall body strength that we all need. As I work with professional athletes in my own practice, I have come to respect the essential role these foods play in a fatigue-free diet for *all* of my patients.

Like fiber, complex carbohydrates keep your energy and emotional levels high, eliminating the energy peaks and valleys that set off the destructive binge-eating cycle, while satisfying the biological cravings that drive us to eat those foods. Both fiber and complex carbohydrates work like a biological insurance policy covering the dangerous, destructive eating patterns that make us fat in the first place.

Foods like pasta and whole grains also help you lose weight by replacing a large amount of fat in your diet. By cutting fat and increasing fiber and complex carbohydrates, you are really making nutritional sense. The energy that we derive from complex carbohydrates is produced in a "time-release" form—that is, these nutrients are burned slowly by the body and are safely and gradually transformed into energy. In contrast, fats and sugar give you a quick energy fix which makes you want to eat more and more. As we all know, food in excess of our energy requirements is stored within the body in the form of unhealthy, disfiguring fat.

Finally, complex carbohydrates are full of the essential vitamins and minerals you need to keep your immune system healthy. They offer vitamins A, B, C, D, and E, a whole complement of vital minerals, and many of the amino acids your body needs. In many ways, they are a "one-stop shop" for many of the crucial nutrients I discuss later in this book, and an efficient way to make sure you get enough of these nutrients in your diet.

Because of the clear value of these carbohydrates in our

health, the recipes in this book take into account what we know about how they work, and how you can use them to build your immune health at the same time as you lower your weight.

CHAPTER SIX

Hidden Food Sensitivities— Immunity's Achilles' Heel

WE HAVE already seen that it is crucial to provide your body with the building blocks necessary to the constant renewal of your immune system. You now know about the immune-fat connection and realize that you must lose the excess weight that destroys immune power.

However, there is one more, very subtle way that what you eat can affect your immune power. The problem is called *masked* or *hidden food sensitivities,* or simply *food allergies*. It is your immune system's Achilles' heel—its secret vulnerability. You may be eating yourself into serious immune weakness without realizing it.

Each of us has specific sensitivities to certain foods which can actually damage those trusty immune soldiers, the lymphocytes. If you looked through a microscope you would be able to see immune cells swell, slow down, and finally explode as they contact these food toxins. In a very real way, some foods are engaged in biological warfare against the very cells essential to our health. When you sit down to dinner, you may, without knowing it, be holding the beginning of biological Armageddon on your fork.

Oddly enough, most people have hidden food sensitivities to the very foods that appear most nourishing and healthy. Allergies to wheat, corn, and dairy products are so common that at least one of these afflicts almost every American. Yeast, sugar, coffee, eggs, and soy products are also common villains.

YOUR IMMUNE FINGERPRINT

Food sensitivities can be as varied as the range of foods we eat, but *each person's specific food sensitivities are unique*. One person may be sensitive to wheat, sugar, picked foods, and dairy products; another to barley, beets, shellfish, and legumes. We can now actually see, by means of sophisticated laboratory techniques, how these foods can destroy our immune cells. It is ironic that it has taken the most up-to-date cell physiology research to show us the biological truth in the old adage, "one man's meat is another man's poison."

Sensitivities are so specific that even siblings raised together, eating the same foods, can develop individual food sensitivities. There are, however, different degrees of sensitivities. Some foods cause only slight damage to a few white blood cells, while others cause massive destruction, killing hundreds of thousands of these cells. Our sensitivities are so personal, in fact, that they make up a sort of biochemical fingerprint—particular, distinctive, and unique. However, unlike fingerprints, these patterns can change over time.

Dr. Theron Randolph, the Chicago physician who is recognized as the founder of our modern science of food allergies, found that we may acquire or lose sensitivities depending on how often we are exposed to a given food. Once, he explains, nature regulated what we ate because most food was seasonal. In the past, we ate what was available, and as the array of fruits and vegetables changed with the seasons, there was an automatic, steady rotation of our diet, so that it was not possible to overdose on a small set of foods.

But modern distribution and mass industrial food production have made most foods available to us year-round. This means that we now have plenty of time to get used to, and overdose on, various foods. No wonder more and more food allergies are being diagnosed, with more people suffering from the effects.

Does this apply to everybody? You bet. You can be sure that you have several major food sensitivities you don't even recognize. Among more than three thousand patients, I have never found *one* whose blood tests did not show a reaction to at least one previously unknown food item. Dr. Randolph estimates that for every one allergy that we *do* recognize in our diet, at least two remain hidden.

TRACKING DOWN YOUR DANGER FOODS

Obviously, it is crucial to have accurate tests for food sensitivities. Most traditional allergists use scratch tests, which involves giving the patient scores of tiny scratches on the back. Then various food extracts are introduced into the skin and the reaction is measured. Unfortunately, the test is time-consuming and often fails to point up hidden food sensitivities. Often, one reaction hides another, or the tests fail to pick up a powerful allergy to a certain food.

Another kind of test is the sublingual test, where potent extracts of food products are put under the tongue. There they are absorbed quickly and the patient is carefully observed for signs of sensitivity reaction. In my experience this type of testing is also time-consuming, and although it is symptom-specific, it too fails to indicate some hidden food intolerances.

Cytotoxic testing is a valuable tool in screening patients for food sensitivities. The test can be done quickly in the laboratory using only one blood sample from each patient, so there is no unnecessary evoking of possible allergic reactions. The test uses a drop of blood which is then exposed to various food extracts. By observing the patient's white blood cells react to different food extracts, hundreds of foods can be tested quickly and efficiently for their immo-toxic potential. I have had superb results using this test to evaluate thousands of patients.

By far the surest, most reliable test is the isolation test. Here, patients are put into a hospital environment where everything—air, water, food, chemicals—can be controlled to be absolutely nonallergenic. This lets patients start with a clean slate. Then, one by one, particular foods are reintroduced and the physician observes the reactions. Because the patient's entire environment is so tightly controlled, this is the best and most accurate way to test for sensitivities. Unfortunately, the unwieldy complexity of this kind of testing makes it prohibitively expensive and time-consuming. The isolation test is reserved for only the most severe sufferers.

Because the "remove and reintroduce" principle is the most accurate and effective means of identifying allergies that we know, I have simplified it and adapted it for the Immune Power Diet. Here, for the first time, is a program for those of us who want to best identify our hidden food sensitivities but can't afford to check into a hospital for two months to do so. The program I outline in the next chapter is a practical version of isolation testing. It offers a realistic, do-it-yourself way you can use these same accurate principles to measure your own food sensitivities.

FOOD SENSITIVITIES AND YOUR HEALTH

I've explained what hidden food sensitivities do to your cells, which means that every one of your immune cells that self-destructs from a food sensitivity is one less immune soldier fighting for your health.

The food you savor at lunch may have damaged or killed tens or even hundreds of thousands of immune cells by midafternoon, resulting in less vigilant immune surveillance, a slower immune response, and a less aggressive immune attack. Of course, your immune defenses keep an ample reserve. Obviously, no *single meal* can do so much damage that you would suddenly be left vulnerable to flu. Often, the effects of hidden food sensitivities aren't even immediately obvious, but they do take an insidious toll.

They do their damage subtly, sapping your strength and vitality. The immune-weakened person grows slowly more sluggish, starts losing vitality, energy, and sexual drive, and the aging process is accelerated, resulting in premature wrinkles and skin problems.

Hidden food sensitivites are also associated with a tremendous range of physical symptoms. I have treated patients suffering from chronic arthritis, fatigue, debilitating headaches, ulcers, skin, and nerve problems. Food sensitivities are known to cause heart palpitations, nausea, vomiting, asthma, dizziness, ear and throat infections, glandular imbalances, muscle aches and pains, rashes, swelling of feet and hands, and abdominal cramps. Because the immune system is so far-reaching, every organ system is touched by the immune imbalances that food sensitivities cause.

FREQUENT FOOD SENSITIVITY SYMPTOMS

Head and Upper Respiratory Tract

Headaches, dizziness, feeling faint, runny nose, blocked nasal passages and sinuses, eyes watering, earache, trouble hearing, throbbing or ringing in the ear, sore throat, chronic ear, eye or throat infections, bleeding gums, itchy eyes and ears, canker sores.

Chest and Stomach

Feeling of fullness in chest, asthma, congestion or fluid in the lungs, persistent coughs, hoarseness, palpitations, rapid heart rate, nausea, vomiting, cramps, gas and flatulence, diarrhea, constipation, stomach feels heavy and bloated long after meals.

Psychological Symptoms

Confusion, lethargy, fatigue, aggression, irritability, hyperactivity, anxiety, depression, crying easily, inability to concentrate, trouble sleeping, sudden sleepiness soon after meals.

Skin Problems

Red spots, rashes, dermatitis, eczema, hives, itching.

Extremities

Weakness in limbs, sore muscles, miscellaneous muscular aches and pains, joint pains, swelling (edema) of feet, ankles, and hands.

Miscellaneous Symptoms

Chronic fatigue, urgency of urination, excessive hunger, rapid or significant changes in weight.

CEREBRAL ALLERGIES:
EMOTIONS IN TURMOIL

Allergic reactions can also be extremely damaging if they affect the brain. These are the *cerebral allergies*, which can create devastating emotional results. I have seen food sensitivities in my patients create a wide range of psychological symptoms: lethargy, anxiety, loss of appetite or sex drive, insomnia, incapacitating depression, and hyperactivity.

Severe sensitivities can precipitate crying jags, raging aggressive behavior, slurred speech, or irritability. I would like to know just how many thousands of people find themselves labeled neurotics and psychotics simply because their doctors don't know how to diagnose the subtle food sensitivities that are causing such emotional havoc.

That was what brought Audrey to my office. Audrey was only twenty-three when she and her new husband, Eric, moved to Manhattan. At first, everything had been wonderful. They each enjoyed their new jobs—he as a hospital administrator, she as a buyer for a department store. Their first year had been a whirl of settling into their first apartment, starting new jobs, and making new friends. Their lives were full and busy, but happy.

About a year later, Audrey noticed things starting to change. At first, she felt more tired and cranky than her usual cheery self. Going out at night with friends became more a chore than a joy. She was not quite able to focus on her job—her attention would wander, and she found the quality of her work slipping.

They both decided the time had come for a vacation and went to Mexico for two weeks. But there, things got worse instead of better. "It seemed like I spent the whole time nagging at Eric for every little thing. He'd misplace bus tickets, and I'd explode. He'd take a picture, and I'd get sulky. I spent that whole trip fuming, angry with Eric and with myself. I hated myself for doing it, and I knew I wasn't being much fun, but couldn't stop.''

Back in New York, the situation became worse yet. Audrey started having crying fits in the middle of the day at work. She became clinically depressed—she had no energy or real sense of enjoyment or push.

Meanwhile, Eric's job was going well. He'd been promoted and was now directing a whole section of the hospital. Yet because of her erratic moods, Audrey's work suffered, and she saw others get promotions she felt she should have. After four months of this, she had come to the end of her rope.

"I felt everything I'd worked for—my marriage and my job—dissolving. New York was closing in on me.''

Her doctor sent her to me for a series of food allergy tests. She seemed a likely candidate for food sensitivity problems. Her fair skin and strawberry blond hair suggested that she might well be allergy-prone, but more importantly, the range of her psychological symptoms— depression, mood swings, behavior disturbances, hopelessness—were the kind of broad symptoms food sensitivities are known to cause. Sure enough, her test reports came back checkered with positive results: wheat, milk, corn, beets, celery, lettuce, citrus fruits, legumes, beef, and shellfish were associated with severe reactions, and weaker sensitivities to a score of other foods were documented.

Audrey went on a special Immune Power Diet, geared to removing her toxic foods and rebuilding her immune system. Within two months, her psychological symptoms had completely disappeared. She was again full of energy, happy, and making up for lost time at work. Her boss had even commented on the change. The happiest was her husband, Eric, who accompanied her on her final office visit. "I was beginning to wonder if I'd ever see again the wonderful, bright person I married," he said. "Thanks for giving her back to me!"

I have seen hundreds of Audreys. All of these patients, once they identify their danger foods and carefully eliminate them from their diet, find their mental state much improved. I hear patients say "I'd forgotten how wonderful it felt to have a restful night's sleep," or "It's been years since I had really let loose and laughed with all my soul."

BATTLE OF THE BINGE: FOOD SENSITIVITIES AT WORK

One of the most devastating effects of food sensitivities is compulsive eating; or food-binge behavior. Binging is defined as explosive, uncontrolled eating far beyond the normal point of satiation. Instead of eating a plate of spaghetti, the binger eats a potful; instead of a bowl of ice cream, several quarts. It is not uncommon for binge eaters to go on uncontrolled, helpless food sprees several times during a week.

This tragic pattern has both physical and psychological roots. *People usually binge on exactly the foods to which they have immune sensitivities*. It is not surprising, then, that the most common food sensitivities—dairy products, wheat, and corn—are represented in the most frequent binge foods: ice cream, pizza, and corn chips.

Although it seems paradoxical that we binge on exactly the foods to which we are most immune-sensitive, research shows that when binge eaters go on a spree, they release a specific type of hormone called *beta endorphins*.

Beta endorphins are the body's own opiate substances, tiny proteins that cause changes in brain chemicals. They are considered to help regulate a wide range of functions, including relief of pain, sexual urges, body temperature, and appetite, as well as psychological activities such as memory, learning, and depression. We also produce a lot of beta endorphins during strenuous exercise, and researchers believe this creates the feelings of well-being and euphoria that many athletes experience—the so-called "runner's high." Because food bingers trigger a release of beta endorphins each time they go on a spree, they are, in effect, giving themselves a "high."

That, in fact, was exactly how Anders, another of my patients, explained it. At first, he said, his friends kidded him about his "addiction" to sweet, sticky desserts, but he began to realize that addiction was no laughing matter. Always a big-boned man (Anders had been a serious football player in college), he now watched as his weight increased by ten, then twenty, and thirty pounds. He would duck out on his lunch hour and make the rounds of bakery and sweet shops in a ten-block radius, buying pastries and wolfing them down before he got to the next store. At first these trips occurred once a week, then accelerated to every other day. "The feeling it gave me was total bliss—the same feeling I used to get after a hard football practice. I'd look forward to my trips a whole day ahead of time like some kind of drug."

It was not until he'd been working with me on the Immune Power Diet that he began to see how very destructive a drug his food binges had been. After two months, his weight dropped twenty-three pounds, and he has set himself a goal of fifteen more. Not surprisingly, his energy and enjoyment of life have flourished as his weight has dropped. But, most important, his attitude has completely reversed. "The very thought of going out on an eating spree now seems alien, almost comical. I can't imagine how I ever used to do it. When I think of what I used to shovel in . . . ugh!"

The binging syndrome isn't all physiological. Dr. Leslie-Jane Maynard, a clinical psychologist noted for her work with compulsive eaters, has shown that binging has strong psychological roots. Dr. Maynard's research with hundreds of patients has shown that compulsive, or "binge," eating results when people don't know how to handle the pressures of their lives. When stress levels get out of control, a food binge works like a safety valve to relieve anxiety momentarily. She has also found that binge eaters actually go into what she calls "binge narcosis" after an eating spree. They fall into a trance-like state, similar to that observed with many narcotic drugs.

Obviously, the worse emotional shape you are in—because of the depression, lethargy, and psychological torment that food sensitivities can cause—the more you binge on food. Conversely, the better you feel about yourself and your life, the less need you have to plunge into destructive eating episodes.

Both at the physical level of measurable brain chemistry, and at the psychological level, binges are a destructive cycle of addiction, a complex physical and psychological conspiracy caused by an immune imbalance.

WHAT'S AHEAD:
POSITIVE IMMUNE HEALTH

In this chapter, I wanted to give you a sense of the wide range of problems food sensitivities can cause. I suspect that many of them may be problems that you, your friends, or family may be having, but never knew were tied to your diet. The rest of the book is dedicated to doing something about this immune imbalance.

Obviously, if you ever hope to achieve truly strong

immune health, the first step is removing those food toxins that are doing so much damage. That's the first part of the three-pronged Immune Power Diet approach. In Section II, you'll find a detailed, step-by-step program for identifying which of the many foods constitute the Achilles' heel of your immune system. I will give you a detailed diet plan whereby you can remove these food intolerances from your diet as you break away from food binging, and also stop the severe damage these foods have done to your immune system.

Section III will show you how to assess your immune status and rebuild your immune system with an individualized plan of vitamin, mineral, and amino acid supplementation. Then you will be ready to build your immune power life-style plan, eating those foods that work for your immune system and supplementing them as necessary so that your immune system can work its best for you.

CHAPTER SEVEN

Your Living Laboratory

NOW THAT you know the damage that food allergies can do to your immune health, the time has come to put that knowledge to work for you.

In this chapter, I will show you how to identify which of the foods you now eat that are hazardous to your immune health. The first step towards superb immune fitness—and the glowing health that goes with it—is to REMOVE these danger foods from your diet.

Unfortunately, that's not easy. You can't find your personal answers in a book or on a chart. No laboratory tests on white mice can reveal your particular reactions to foods. The only one with answers for you is you. That means that you must use your own body as a living laboratory and conduct your own systematic tests of your reactions to various foods.

First, I will show you how to ELIMINATE the foods that might damage your immune fitness. Next, you will learn how to CHALLENGE your body by reintroducing certain foods to determine which are *your* problem foods. Once you have identified your danger foods, you can maintain your immune health by either gradually desensitizing yourself to these foods, or if that is impossible, removing them totally from your diet.

PHASE I: ELIMINATE

The goal of this phase is to eliminate the foods that are the most common cause of immune imbalance. We are going to use a fundamental principle of modern science: to see the effect of something you must isolate it.

Most of us have several food allergies of varying severity, that often overlap. Sometimes, one allergy masks the effects of another. Sometimes, the reverse occurs and, in what physicians call *potentiation,* two sensitivities combine to create more severe symptoms than either food allergy alone would create. Trying to unravel such overlapping allergies without isolating each food sensitivity is like trying to feel a light breeze in the middle of a typhoon. In order to see clearly which way the breeze is blowing, you have to calm the "immune typhoon."

Phase One quiets this turbulence by removing the foods which are the most likely sources of your immune problems. This diet has been very carefully designed to make your body eliminate the foods that damage your immune efficiency. The 21-day Elimination diet, in Part II, allows those interlocking and overlapping immune responses to subside so that your immune system becomes relatively quiet.

Many of my patients ask how any one diet can remove all the foods that endanger a person. The answer is, of course, that it can't—not 100 percent. But research has proven again and again that a select group of seven major food culprits create the overwhelming majority of food sensitivities. I find these so often in my medical practice that I have come to call them the Sinister Seven Target Foods.

THE SINISTER SEVEN TARGET FOODS

The seven foods are those which, in my clinical experience, create immune damage in the overwhelming majority of patients. Together, they account for about 85 percent of the food reactions I have seen in thousands of my patients. Even more important, the Sinister Seven are those foods I have found closely linked to food binging and excess weight. In order of frequency, they are:

Cow's milk products	Corn
Wheat	Soy products
Brewer's and Baker's Yeast	Cane sugar
Eggs	

Although these foods are the worst offenders, they are by no means the only problem foods. Any food can cause a negative reaction, depending on the individual biochemical makeup of the person affected. Some particular foods and food groups even seem linked to very particular symptoms.

SPECIFIC SYMPTOMS FROM FOODS

- Foods such as coffee, cocoa, and chocolate, which all contain caffeine, often create the particular symptom of headaches in my patients.
- Foods such as tomatoes, eggplants, bell peppers, white onions, potatoes, paprika, zucchini, and squash seem tied to a variety of arthritic and joint symptoms.
- Dairy foods such as milk, cream, butter, yogurt, and all kinds of cheeses cause particularly troublesome

responses in the form of asthma as well as a number of gastrointestinal symptoms including cramps, gas, bloating, diarrhea, and constipation.

- Common citrus fruits—oranges, lemons, grapefruits, tangerines, and limes—are linked to a wide range of traditional allergic symptoms including hives, wheezing, and headaches.

You won't find these links between food-specific reactions and immunocompetence reported elsewhere; food sensitivities are not yet commonly considered immune reactions. In fact, it may be years until this association is fully documented. However, my findings, which are based on extensive clinical observation and testing of my patients, can begin to work for you today by means of the Immune Power Diet.

Not only does this diet program remove all of the Sinister Seven, as well as the other most common danger foods from your diet, it also removes a whole range of additives, preservatives, and chemicals often found in foods. Thousands of these additives, including MSG (monosodium glutamate), BHT, polysorbate, disodium inosinate, and sodium benzoate, are used today. Not only do many of these chemicals have their own toxic effect on immune health but they magnify toxic responses caused by other foods. The result is an even bigger assault on our immune cells.

EMBARKING ON PHASE ONE

Section II includes easy recipes for many commonly purchased processed foods such as broths, mayonnaise, salad dressings, spaghetti sauce, and sorbets that avoid potentially harmful additives. Now you can make your own versions of these foods, free of additives, preservatives, and chemicals. In section II, you will also find the detailed day-to-day diet. It is a clear, straightforward plan: 3 meals a day plus snacks for 21 days, based on a 4-day rotation cycle. My experience shows that twenty-one days is enough time to clear food toxins effectively from the body, and produce a strong immune foundation.

Many patients prefer to stay on it longer because this is the stage when most patients lose most of their weight. I have often seen patients, delighted and astounded at having lost ten to fifteen pounds in three weeks, decide to continue on the diet, and every one of them has achieved an even more impressive weight loss. If you have a truly significant amount of weight to lose, I encourage you to continue beyond the 21-day period.

If you do want to continue this intensive phase longer than the 21 days, simply begin again at Day 1 after the 21-day cycle is finished. You may then continue for four, five, six weeks, or longer. (Many patients have stayed on the diet for several months.) I suggest you consult your physician if you plan to stay on the diet longer than the 21-day cycle.

The Immune Power Diet is carefully designed to be quite safe and healthy over a long period of time. However, there is one rule: *you must complete the cycle of any four-day rotation you start*. This is extremely important. Do not stop half-way through a four-day cycle, because that can upset the nutrient balance that makes this diet so extraordinarily effective. Substitutions for a known food sensitivity or allergy are recommended. Follow the diet as precisely as possible. The more scrupulously you adhere to its balanced program, the more, and more rapid, benefit you will feel.

WITHDRAWAL:
THE SIGN IT'S WORKING

I will tell you up front that the first week is the most demanding period of the entire Immune Power Diet program. Most people experience a series of withdrawal symptoms during the first few days as the body rids itself of accumulated toxins. Biologists call this process *detoxification*.

Here is a description of what happens. Your immune system doesn't recognize at first that the toxins it is so used to fighting are no longer there, so it mounts its usual furious response. The symptoms you feel indicate that your body has, indeed, grown accustomed to using its immune power against the foods that you eat. Physicians have long recognized this phenomenon when toxins like cigarettes, alcohol, heroin and other addictive drugs are withdrawn, but only recently have we understood that this same effect can be associated with foods.

When I explained the diet to Linden, she told me she didn't "believe in" withdrawals. She had come for help with headaches that were growing more and more frequent and severe. Neither her family doctor nor a neurologist had found anything wrong so she had come to me for a food sensitivity test.

Because her tests showed a strong reaction to citrus fruits and some spices, I put her on a diet that eliminated these foods. Two days after she had begun the diet I got an urgent phone call: "My headaches are back, throbbing worse than ever. Plus, I feel dizzy and weak. Last night, I felt sweaty and nervous, I could hardly sleep. What's going on here?"

I wasn't surprised. Often, the stronger the food sensitivity, the more severe the immune response when the offender is eliminated. I told her all that, gave her some suggestions for reducing the headaches, and encouraged her to stay with it. "All right Doctor, I'll give it two more days—but if it isn't better then . . ." she trailed off.

I didn't get a call two days later, or even four. Finally, two weeks later, she came into the office. "You know, those headaches stopped the very same day. I haven't had one since—and that's the first time I could say that in years!" She went on to explain that she felt like a new woman, full of energy and sleeping well. "And, best of all," she beamed, "I've lost twelve pounds!"

Not everybody experiences the strong withdrawal that Linden had. For those who do, symptoms can be quite severe, taking the form of severe headaches, profound tiredness and lethargy, stomach upset, joint and muscle pains, acne and skin rashes. Psychological reactions are equally common: you may find yourself irritable, tense, nervous, have profound mood swings, or be unable to sleep well.

Well, believe it or not, these unpleasant symptoms are good news on two counts. First, they *are clear signs that the Elimination diet is working*. These are the signal that your immune system is actively clearing out the damage done to it by food toxins. For many people, the worse the symptoms during this period, the greater the benefit they feel later. Remind yourself that every symptom is *proof* of how much your body needed a good immune tune-up, and proof of how much benefit you will get from the Immune Power Diet.

As for the other good news, it's like the old joke about taking off tight shoes: cheer up, it's soon over! By the end of the first week—or ten days, at most—withdrawal symptoms usually disappear.

WITHDRAWAL TIP

If you do experience particularly severe withdrawal symptoms in the first week of the diet, here's a tip that has helped many of my patients. Take one 1000-milligram tablet of vitamin C every three hours, up to six each day. *It is essential to drink a lot of water when taking this much vitamin C.* If you experience gastric discomfort or diarrhea, cut the dose in half.

After the withdrawal period, your real payoff begins. Now you begin to enjoy the benefits of a clean, finely-tuned immune system. This is the point when most of my patients see a dramatic drop in any symptoms they might have had. You can look for improvements in a whole range of areas. Headaches and stomach problems disappear, swelling, puffiness and edema soon resolve, a host of minor aches and pains in your joints and muscles may clear up. Most people find themselves sleeping better, awakening refreshed. Anxiety and depression start lifting, and with them go the abrupt mood swings. You can look forward to your whole being feeling lighter, clearer, more full of energy and vitality. Your stamina and endurance will probably improve. In short, you can start enjoying all the health benefits of a streamlined, robust immune system. And remember your trillion immune cells? Listen close, and you'll almost hear them humming happily . . .

PHASE II: REINTRODUCTION

Now you are ready for the second, or Reintroduction phase of the Immune Power Diet—the stage in which you systematically reintroduce specific foods into your diet to learn if any of these foods cause reactions. You will have become vastly more sensitive to the signals your body is sending you, and it is crucial in this phase, to listen acutely to those signals.

Most of us aren't in the habit of listening closely to the information our bodies are constantly sending us. A twinge here, an ache there, slight soreness or creakiness in a joint, a rumbling in your tummy, a slight fever . . . we get hundreds of such hints every day. Unfortunately, we rarely pay attention until they get so loud—a strained back, say, or a raging temperature—that we can no longer ignore them.

LISTENING TO YOUR BODY

Try this exercise. Take a moment to feel what your body is telling you right now. You're probably sitting in a chair as you read this. Feel your lower back. Is there muscle strain? Is your neck relaxed or tense? Do your eyes ache just a bit? Does your stomach feel tight or heavy?

You must now be a careful observer of the signals your body sends as you *challenge* it by reintroducing, one at a time, the Sinister Seven foods. These challenge symptoms can take the same variety of forms as the food allergy symptoms I listed earlier—which makes sense because they are one and the same.

But whatever form they take, you will recognize them when they happen. You must assume that anything wrong you feel during this period is due to the danger foods you have eaten—particularly if you have not experienced the symptoms in the preceding 21-day elimination phase.

Follow this pattern throughout the Reintroduction phase of the diet: *every other day* eat the target food from the Sinister Seven for that day. Eat it three times. You can use the recipes and serving suggestions I provide in section II, or not, depending on your taste. But the essential thing is to eat this particular food *three times* on those days. This will be a sufficient amount to elicit any response you might have. Challenge for one day, observe for one day, then change to another target food from the Sinister Seven list.

Continue this way, introducing a new food every forty-eight hours, and observing your reactions, until you have reintroduced all of the Sinister Seven foods back into your diet. At the end of that two-week period, you will be able to pinpoint the foods you are specifically sensitive to. You will have a list of those foods which cause severe reactions, which cause weak reactions, and which are harmless.

YOUR PERSONAL 14-DAY REINTRODUCTION TIMETABLE AND LOG

Day	Sinister Seven Food	Symptoms
1	Corn	
2	——	
3	Soy Products	
4	——	
5	Cane Sugar	
6	——	
7	Eggs	
8	——	
9	Baker's and Brewer's Yeast	
10	——	
11	Cow's Milk	
12	——	
13	Wheat	
14	——	

You will now be able to customize your diet to avoid your own immune danger foods. But the Immune Power Diet is completely flexible so that it fits perfectly with *your* own immune needs. Obviously, if you observe a consistent problem with a certain food, even though it may not be frequent or common danger food for others, you must avoid it.

Depending on the degree of improvement in your overall health, you may decide that you want to try isolating other, less common danger foods you feel might be causing problems. You now have the tools to do it. Now that you have achieved a high level of immune efficiency you can use the same eliminate/reintroduce principle whenever you want to test for immune-toxic responses you may have to other specific foods.

PHASE III: MAINTAIN

Phase III shows you how to maintain this finely tuned immune system. By relieving your immune cells of the burden caused by immune-damaging foods in Phase I and Phase II, you made it possible for the system to function at its peak force. The goal of this final phase, *maintenance*, is to keep you at this peak of immune health and performance by building good immune habits into your life.

The key to this is practicality and flexibility. After all, no diet, no matter how healthy, is useful if you can't stay on it. If it is so restrictive that it won't work in the real world, you will be unable to maintain the advances in immune health you have achieved.

MAINTENANCE AND MODERATION: THE FOUR-DAY PLAN

The maintenance phase works because it is so adaptable. There are no hard and fast rules here; it is basically an overall philosophy of how you should eat. That philosophy follows the one first enunciated at the height of ancient Greek civilization millennia ago. They called it *syphrosyne*, which translates as *moderation*, or the Golden Mean.

Three thousand years later, the rule still applies. In many cases of food intolerance you can start eating your danger foods again, *if you do so in moderation*. (Note: If you have a severe allergy, you should not try to reintroduce a food.) Suppose you have discovered a wide variety of food sensitivities, or that certain of the foods which you are hypersensitive to are the very foods you love and can't imagine cutting out altogether. Does this mean you have to live like a cloistered monk, completely denying yourself foods that give you true enjoyment? Is that the dreary price of immune health?

Absolutely not! Over fifty years ago, pioneer allergists discovered that by eating danger foods no more than *once every four days,* the body avoids the negative responses it otherwise would suffer, because the limited frequency gives the body the chance to absorb these foods. This four-day limit is widely recognized in the field of food allergies, and has been confirmed in clinical experience the world over. In a science where little is well-understood, this is one principle which is widely upheld and accepted.

Using this four-day plan, you can keep your food intolerances well under control because your immune system is now so much stronger than it was when you began the Immune Power Diet. When you eliminated the immune overdose of danger foods, you did two things. First, you actually reduced the severity of the response itself. Second, you let the body rebuild its own strength. By breaking the sensitivity cycle, you became more resistant, and less sensitive, to *moderate* exposures to these foods.

True, sensitivity responses differ in strength, ranging from sub-clinical reactions you don't even recognize to full-blown emergency allergic responses. That means that some of your most severe sensitivities may still create symptoms, but many of the others will disappear, so that you can eat those foods moderately on a four-day cycle.

By following this simple philosophy of food rotation, you will continue to use your diet to build strong health. Chapter 9 contains a sample Maintenance Diet menu for one week, and a variety of delicious recipes that are especially well-suited to the program. But these are given to show you the possibilities of the program. You will undoubtedly want to create your own menu plans and recipes and I encourage you to do so, provided you continue to use the rotation principle and other sound nutritional guidelines described in Section II.

THE ART OF BEING GOOD TO YOURSELF

By far the most important part of the maintenance philosophy has nothing to do with the biochemistry of food intolerances—it's in your head. In order to make the Immune Power Diet really work for you, you need to learn how to do your body the kinds of favors that help it, instead of the "favors" that hurt it.

We are all conditioned by advertisements and the huge junk food industry that being "kind" to ourselves means satisfying all of our immediate food wants and cravings. They have told us that it's a favor to our body to indulge in all sorts of cheap food thrills: snacking on foods that are sweet, salty, full of refined sugar, chemicals, and artificial flavoring.

But such "favors" are illusory and short-lived. I agree that we all need to treat ourselves, and be kind to ourselves—but I mean real favors and true kindness. In the Immune Power Diet, I ask you to do yourself a real, lasting, and profound favor: give your body what it needs to *support and renew your immune health-keeper*.

I have found that my patients who show the most spectacular progress, who lose the most weight and gain the most in health, vitality, and enjoyment of life, have one thing in common: a positive attitude.

They don't seem to spend much time worrying about those things they *can't* eat. That's not their focus at all. Instead, they revel in the glowing feeling of knowing they are fueling themselves with immune-positive foods. They see the diet not as a foe, but as an ally.

One of my patients, Karen, put it best two months after she started the program. "Dr. Berger, all I knew in the beginning was that you wanted me to make big changes in what I eat every day, and I wasn't convinced. But I now see it wasn't about that at all. It was really about cleaning out my whole life, from top to bottom. Why didn't you say so?"

Since she said that, I've always had patients pose themselves the right question before the start the diet. *Don't* ask yourself if you want to make a big change in *what you eat,* ask yourself if you want to make a big change in *how you feel.*

SECTION II

The Immune Power Diet

**Diet and recipes prepared by
Mary Beth Clark,
The Food Consulting Group, and
The Mary Beth Clark Cooking School**

I wish to thank my parents, Dr. Eugene V. Clark and Rita Ann Clark, R. N., for their expert medical advice and constant support, and my husband and best friend, Dr. B. Alva Schoomer, for his wise counsel and tasting of countless meals. To my assistant, Mary Dalessandro, I extend my gratitude for the many hours of typing, editing, and testing as well as her sound advice; and, also, my thanks to Lara Hopfl.

I also wish to thank the editors, Michaela Hamilton and Molly Allen, for their support throughout the writing of this book.

CHAPTER EIGHT

Eating for Immune Power

THE NEXT PAGES contain the simple, easy-to-follow diet that has worked for so many of my patients. You'll find everything here that you need to quite literally eat your way to health. It lays out a clear, 21-day plan that shows you, step by step, how to detoxify your immune system, a two-week gradual reintroduction phase, a maintenance diet for men and women, and a set of patient-tested recipes to help you stay healthy and thin. You may want to go back and read chapter 7 if you have any questions about the diet. But if you don't, here are a few basic principles to keep in mind.

This entire diet is based on the magic number "4." The four-day rotation principle ensures that you do not eat the same food more than once every four days in order to prevent food sensitivities. This underlying principle is built into the elimination, reintroduction, and maintenance menus in this section.

Be sure to eat each of the three meals and snacks per day that are called for in the diets. Skipping meals will only make you overly hungry, and encourage overeating later. The diet plans have been designed to satisfy your appetite as well as your nutritional needs. Of course, if you have already identified a food sensitivity or allergy, you will want to make appropriate substitutions using foods that are safe for you.

When selecting a piece of fruit for the diet menus, select average size fruit, which means small to medium size, depending on season and availability.

The menus have been designed to fit into your personal life-style. Try the recipes in this section—they are delicious and unusual. If you wish to branch out after you follow my menus you can, but just remember *the four-day rule*.

When you plan your own menus (after completing the 21-day plan), try to use at leat four of each kind of food. I happen to like fruit juices, so I enjoy a different kind on each day for four consecutive days. The same applies with the four types of main courses from the different food groups: shellfish, fish, poultry, and meat, as well as herbal teas, and grains. Of course, no rule says you *must* eat the same food every four days. If you want to eat some foods only once a week, or once every two weeks, that's even better. The more foods you come to enjoy, the less often you'll eat any one food item. But remember, you can't have the same food any more *often* than *once in four days*.

Obviously, there will be times you will depart from this rule. If the Queen of Sheba should invite you for high tea and crumpets, you'd hardly want to turn her down simply because you ate crumpets yesterday. Even if you don't get calls from the Queen that often, there will probably be occasions when you'll have to break the four-day rule. You may be someone who eats out often, or travels a good deal. (If so, you will find many good tips for these circumstances in the Eating Out and Travel sections in this chapter.)

So don't worry, if you occasionally depart from the four-day schedule, the sky won't cave in. Do the best you can, keeping the rotation principle in mind. That way, you will still be building on the principles of immune health by generally eliminating the Sinister Seven Target Foods and rotating foods as much as possible.

CHAPTER NINE

Menus and Recipes

THE 21-DAY ELIMINATION DIET MENU

Instructions for preparing starred dishes will be found in the recipe section (pages 127–234)

WEEK 1 DAY 1

BREAKFAST I   Nectarine (1), apricots (2), or tangelo (1)
Boiled Pearl Barley* (½ cup)
Cranberry juice (1 cup)
Coffee substitute or herbal tea

OR

BREAKFAST II†   Nectarines (2), apricots (4), or tangelos (2)
Cranberry juice (1 cup)
Coffee substitute or herbal tea

LUNCH   Tabouleh Salad* (1¼ cups) or beef barley soup (2 cups)
Mineral water or seltzer

DINNER   Broiled red snapper or bass (4 ounces)
Broiled Sweet Red Pepper* (1)
Romaine lettuce salad (unlimited) with diced cucumber (¼ cup) and diced tomato (½ cup)
Tomato Juice Salad Dressing* (unlimited)
Nectarine (1) or apricots (3)
Coffee substitute, herbal tea, mineral water, or seltzer

SNACK   Fresh goat cheese (1 ounce)

*Recipes appears in recipe section.
†If selecting Breakfast II, serve the Boiled Pearl Barley (½ cup) at lunch or dinner, or as a snack, and eliminate 1 fruit serving at lunch or dinner.

WEEK 1 DAY 2

BREAKFAST I   Strawberries (½ cup)
                   Oatmeal (½ cup) or oatcake crackers (2)
                   Fresh unsweetened orange juice (1 cup)
                   Coffee substitute or herbal tea

OR

BREAKFAST II†   Strawberries (1 cup)
                   Fresh unsweeened orange juice (1 cup)
                   Coffee substitute or herbal tea

LUNCH   Tuna (3½-ounce can, water-packed, or 4
                       ounces fresh broiled)
                   or Broiled chicken (4 ounces)
                   Steamed green beans (1 cup)
                   Steamed potatoes (1 cup)
                   Kiwi (1)
                   Mineral water or seltzer

DINNER   Parsnip and Leek Soup* (1 cup)
                   Broiled chicken (4 ounces)
                   Sautéed Okra* or steamed green beans
                       (1 cup)
                   Swiss chard or endive salad (unlimited)
                   Citrus Salad dressing* (unlimited)
                   Strawberries (½ cup)
                   Coffee substitute, herbal tea, mineral
                   . water, or seltzer

SNACK   Orange or kiwi (1)

*Recipe appears in recipe section.
†If selecting Breakfast II, serve the oatmeal (½ cup) or oatcake crackers (2) at lunch
or dinner, or as a snack, and eliminate 1 fruit serving at lunch or dinner.

WEEK 1 DAY 3

BREAKFAST I   Banana (½)
Puffed rice cereal (½ cup), rice cake (1),
or rice crackers (4)
Unsweetened apple juice (½ cup)
Coffee substitute or herbal tea

OR

BREAKFAST II†   Banana (1)
Unsweetened apple juice (½ cup)
Coffee substitute or herbal tea

LUNCH   Fruit Plate: Sliced apple (1), sliced banana
(½), and watermelon or Persian melon
cubes (¾ cup)
Mineral water or seltzer

DINNER   Broiled lamb chop (4 ounces)
Stir-Fried Snow Peas with Water Chest-
nuts* (1⅛ cups)
Pureed steamed rutabaga or white turnip
(½ cup)
Boiled Long-Grain Brown Rice* (½ cup)
Baked Apple* (1)
Coffee substitute, herbal tea, mineral
water, or seltzer

SNACK   Rice cake (1) or rice crackers (4)

*Recipe appears in recipe section.
†If selecting Breakfast II, serve the rice cake (1), puffed rice cereal (½ cup), or rice
crackers (4) at lunch or dinner, or as a snack, and eliminate 1 fruit serving at lunch
or dinner.

WEEK 1 DAY 4

BREAKFAST I   Blueberries (½ cup)
                 Puffed millet cereal (1 cup) or Boiled
                     Millet* (½ cup) with 1 tablespoon maple
                     syrup (optional)
                 Fresh unsweetened grapefruit juice (1 cup)
                 Coffee substitute or herbal tea

     OR

BREAKFAST II†   Blueberries (1 cup)
                 Fresh unsweetened grapefruit juice (1 cup)
                 Coffee substitute or herbal tea

LUNCH   Black-eyed peas or pinto beans with thyme
                     (½ cup)
                 or Broiled halibut or swordfish (4 ounces)
                 Steamed vegetable plate: Carrots (1 cup),
                     cauliflower (1 cup), and chickory or
                     escarole (2 cups)
                 Tangerine or peach (1)
                 Mineral water or seltzer

DINNER   Broiled halibut or swordfish (4 ounces)
                 Steamed Asparagus with Tarragon* (1 cup)
                 Steamed cauliflower (½ cup)
                 Chickory or escarole salad (unlimited)
                 Citrus Salad Dressing* (unlimited)
                 Blueberries (½ cup)
                 Coffee substitute, herbal tea, mineral water,
                     or seltzer

SNACK   Carrot juice (1 cup) or
                 Tangerine or peach (1)

---

*Recipe appears in recipe section.
†If selecting Breakfast II, serve the puffed millet cereal (1 cup) or Boiled Millet (½
cup) with 1 tablespoon maple syrup (optional) at lunch or dinner, or as a snack, and
eliminate 1 fruit serving at lunch or dinner.

WEEK 1 DAY 5

BREAKFAST I   Mango or papaya (½)
               Yeast-free 100% rye bread (1 slice), 100%
                 rye crackers (2) or rye cereal (½ cup)
               Coffee substitute or herbal tea

        OR

BREAKFAST II†   Mango or papaya (1)
               Unsweetened grape juice or apricot nectar
                 (1 cup)
               Coffee substitute or herbal tea

LUNCH   Spinach and feta salad: Spinach (unlim-
                 ited), diced cucumber (¼ cup), diced
                 tomato (¼ cup), sliced bermuda or red
                 onion (unlimited), and feta cheese (1
                 ounce)
               Citrus Salad Dressing (unlimited)
               Yeast-free 100% rye bread (1 slice) or
                 100% rye crackers (2)
               or
               Broiled lean ground chuck patty or sliced
                 roast beef (4 ounces)
               Sliced tomato (½ cup)
               Mineral water or seltzer

DINNER   Tomato juice (½ cup) with celery stick (1)
                 and lime wedge
               Broiled lean ground chuck patty or sliced
                 roast beef (4 ounces)
               Steamed brussels sprouts (½ cup)
               Steamed lima beans (½ cup)
               Spinach salad (unlimited)
               Citrus Salad Dressing* (unlimited)
               Grapes (½ cup) or apricots (3)
               Coffee substitute, herbal tea, mineral wa-
                 ter, or seltzer

SNACK   Tomato juice (½ cup) with celery stick (1)
                 and lime wedge or mango or papaya (½)

*Recipe appears in recipe section.
†If selecting Breakfast II, serve the yeast-free 100% rye crackers (2), 100% rye
bread (1 slice), or rye cereal (½ cup) at lunch or dinner, or as a snack, and eliminate
1 fruit serving at lunch or dinner.

WEEK 1 DAY 6

BREAKFAST I   Plums (2) or figs (3)
Boiled Pearl Barley* (½ cup)
Fresh unsweetened orange juice (1 cup)
Coffee substitute or herbal tea

OR

BREAKFAST II†   Plums (4) or figs (6)
Fresh unsweetened orange juice (1 cup)
Coffee substitute or herbal tea

LUNCH   Tuna (3½-ounce can, water-packed, or 4
ounces fresh broiled)
or Broiled chicken (4 ounces)
Steamed green beans or yellow wax beans
(1 cup)
Steamed yellow squash (½ cup)
Watercress salad (unlimited)
Citrus Salad Dressing* (unlimited)
Orange (1)
Mineral water or seltzer

DINNER   Römertopf Roast Chicken with Herbs* (4
ounces)
Steamed green beans or yellow wax beans
(1 cup)
Sautéed zucchini in 1 tablespoon dairy-
free low-fat margarine (½ cup)
Watercress salad (unlimited)
Citrus Salad Dressing* (unlimited)
Figs (2)
Coffee substitute, herbal tea, mineral wa-
ter, or seltzer

SNACK   Plums (2)

*Recipe appears in recipe section.
†If selecting Breakfast II, serve the Boiled Pearl Barley (½ cup) at lunch or dinner,
or as a snack, and eliminate 1 fruit serving at lunch or dinner.

WEEK 1 DAY 7

BREAKFAST I   Unsweetened pineapple (½ cup)
Puffed rice cereal (½ cup), rice cake (1),
   or rice crackers (4)
Coffee substitute or herbal tea

OR
BREAKFAST II†   Unsweetened pineapple (1 cup)
Blackberry or black cherry juice (1 cup)
Coffee substitute or herbal tea

LUNCH   White Bean Salad* (1¼ cups)
or
Sliced roast turkey (4 ounces)
Rice cake (1) or rice crackers (4)
Mineral water or seltzer

DINNER   Sliced roast turkey (4 ounces)
Steamed broccoli (1 cup)
Bibb or Boston lettuce salad (unlimited)
Citrus Salad Dressing* (unlimited)
Boiled Long-Grain Brown Rice* (½ cup)
Pineapple Mousse Sorbet* (1 cup) or un-
   sweetened pineapple (½ cup)
Coffee substitute, herbal tea, mineral wa-
   ter, or seltzer

SNACK   Unsweetened pineapple (½ cup)

*Recipe appears in recipe section.
†If selecting Breakfast II, serve the puffed rice cereal (½ cup), rice cake (1), or rice
crackers (4) at lunch or dinner, or as a snack, and eliminate 1 fruit serving at lunch
or dinner.

WEEK 2 DAY 1

BREAKFAST I   Raspberries (½ cup) or honeydew or can-
taloupe melon (¼)
Oatmeal (½ cup) or oatcake crackers (2)
with 1 tablespoon honey
Guava or passion fruit juice (1 cup)
Coffee substitute or herbal tea

OR
BREAKFAST II†   Raspberries (1 cup) or honeydew or canta-
loupe melon (½)
Guava or passion fruit juice (1 cup)
Coffee substitute or herbal tea

LUNCH   Fruit and cheese plate: Sliced pear (1),
honeydew or cantaloupe melon cubes (1
cup), raspberries (½ cup), and fresh goat
cheese (1 ounce)
Oatcake crackers (2)
or
Broiled red snapper or bass (4 ounces)
Honeydew or cantaloupe melon cubes (1
cup) or guava (1)
Mineral water or seltzer

DINNER   Papillotes*: Red Snapper, Pompano, or Bass
(4 ounces)
Steamed potatoes (1 cup) with chopped
parsley (¼ cup) and 1 tablespoon dairy-
free, low-fat margarine
Arugula salad (unlimited)
Citrus Salad Dressing* (unlimited)
Chinese Steamed Pears* (1)
Coffee substitute, herbal tea, mineral wa-
ter, or seltzer

SNACK   Honeydew or cantaloupe melon (¼) or
guava (1)

---

*Recipe appears in recipe section.
†If selecting Breakfast II, serve the oatmeal (½ cup) or oatcake crackers (2) with 1
tablespoon honey at lunch or dinner, or as a snack, and eliminate 1 fruit serving at
lunch or dinner.

WEEK 2 DAY 2

BREAKFAST I   Unsweetened mandarin orange sections (½ cup)

Buckwheat Groats or Kasha* (½ cup) with 1 tablespoon maple syrup (optional)

Fresh unsweetened grapefruit juice (½ cup)

Coffee substitute or herbal tea

OR

BREAKFAST II†   Unsweetened mandarin orange sections (1 cup)

Fresh unsweetened grapefruit juice (½ cup)

Coffee substitute or herbal tea

LUNCH   Salmon (3¾-ounce can, water packed, or 4 ounces fresh broiled)

or Broiled veal chop (4 ounces)

Steamed peas (½ cup)

Radish sprout, alfalfa sprout, or endive salad (unlimited)

Citrus Salad Dressing* (unlimited)

Mandarin orange sections (½ cup)

Mineral water or seltzer

DINNER   Veal Pojarski* (4 ounces)

Pureed steamed parsnips or rutabaga (½ cup)

Steamed peas (½ cup)

Endive salad (unlimited)

Citrus Salad Dressing* (unlimited)

Grapefruit Sorbet* (1 cup)

Coffee substitute, herbal tea, mineral water, or seltzer

SNACK   Celery sticks (2)

*Recipe appears in recipe section.
†If selecting Breakfast II, serve the Buckwheat Groats or Kasha (½ cup) with 1 tablespoon maple syrup (optional) at lunch or dinner, or as a snack, and eliminate 1 fruit serving at lunch or dinner.

WEEK 2 DAY 3

BREAKFAST I Mango or papaya (½)
Yeast-free 100% rye bread (1 slice), 100% rye crackers (2) or rye cereal (½ cup)
Coffee substitute or herbal tea

OR

BREAKFAST II† Mango or papaya (1)
Unsweetened grape juice or apricot nectar (1 cup)
Coffee substitute or herbal tea

LUNCH Spinach and feta salad: Spinach (unlimited), sliced bermuda or red onion or scallions (unlimited), artichoke hearts (¾ cup), and feta cheese (1 ounce)
Citrus Salad Dressing* (unlimited)
Yeast-free 100% rye bread (1 slice) or 100% rye crackers (2)
or
Sliced roast leg or lamb or broiled lamb chop with rosemary (4 ounces)
Spinach salad (unlimited)
Citrus Salad Dressing* (unlimited)
Mineral water or seltzer

DINNER Sliced roast leg of lamb or broiled lamb chop with rosemary (4 ounces)
Broiled Eggplant* (½)
Steamed cauliflower (½ cup)
Steamed lima beans (½ cup)
Spinach salad (unlimited)
Citrus Salad Dressing* (unlimited)
Mango or papaya (½)
Coffee substitute, herbal tea, mineral water, or seltzer

SNACK Bing cherries or grapes (½ cup)

*Recipe appears in recipe section.
†If selecting Breakfast II, serve the yeast-free 100% rye crackers (2), 100% rye bread (1 slice), or rye cereal (½ cup) at lunch or dinner, or as a snack, and eliminate 1 fruit serving at lunch or dinner.

WEEK 2 DAY 4

BREAKFAST I Peach (1 cup) or tangerines (2)
      Puffed millet cereal (1 cup) or Boiled Millet* (½ cup)
      Unsweetened pineapple juice (1 cup)
      Coffee substitute or herbal tea

OR
BREAKFAST II† Peaches (2 cups) or tangerines (3)
      Unsweetened pineapple juice (1 cup)
      Coffee substitute or herbal tea

LUNCH Sliced roast turkey (4 ounces)
      Steamed beets (1 cup)
      Steamed Carrots with Dill* (1 cup)
      Unsweetened pineapple (1 cup)
      Mineral water or seltzer

DINNER Steamed platter: Flounder, fluke, turbot, sand dab, or sole (4 ounces), asparagus (½ cup), Carrots with Dill* (1 cup)
      Watercress salad (2 cups)
      Citrus Salad Dressing* (unlimited)
      Pineapple Mousse Sorbet* (1 cup) or unsweetened pineapple (½ cup)
      Coffee substitute, herbal tea, mineral water, or seltzer

SNACK Unsweetened pineapple (½ cup)

---

*Recipe appears in recipe section.
†If selecting Breakfast II, serve the puffed millet cereal (1 cup) or Boiled Millet (½ cup) at lunch or dinner, or as a snack, and eliminate 1 fruit serving at lunch or dinner.

WEEK 2 DAY 5

BREAKFAST I
Nectarine (1), apricots (2), or tangelo (1)
Boiled Pearl Barley* (½ cup)
Cranberry juice (1 cup)
Coffee substitute or herbal tea

OR
BREAKFAST II†
Nectarines (2), apricots (4), or tangelos (2)
Cranberry juice (1 cup)
Coffee substitute or herbal tea

LUNCH
Tabouleh Salad* (1¼ cups)
Plum (1)
Mineral water or seltzer

DINNER
Broiled fish and vegetable platter: Blue-fish, tilefish, or perch (4 ounces), green pepper (1), tomato with herbs* (½)
Leaf lettuce salad (unlimited) with diced cucumber (¼ cup)
Tomato Juice Salad Dressing* (unlimited)
Nectarine (1) or apricots (3)
Coffee substitute, herbal tea, mineral water, or seltzer

SNACK
Fresh goat cheese (1 ounce)

*Recipe appears in recipe section.
†If selecting Breakfast II, serve the Boiled Pearl Barley (½ cup) at lunch or dinner, or as a snack, and eliminate 1 fruit serving at lunch or dinner.

WEEK 2 DAY 6

BREAKFAST I   Strawberries (½ cup)
Oatmeal (½ cup) or oatcake crackers (2)
Fresh unsweetened orange juice (1 cup)
Coffee substitute or herbal tea

OR
BREAKFAST II†   Strawberries (1 cup)
Fresh unsweetened orange juice (1 cup)
Coffee substitute or herbal tea

LUNCH   Tuna (3½-ounce can, water packed, or 4
ounces fresh broiled)
or Broiled chicken (4 ounces)
Steamed green beans with marjoram (1
cup)
Steamed potatoes (1 cup)
Kiwi (1)
Mineral water or seltzer

DINNER   Rutabaga and Leek Soup* (1 cup)
Chicken Pojarski* (4 ounces)
Sautéed Okra* or steamed green beans (1
cup)
Swiss chard or endive salad (unlimited)
Citrus Salad Dressing* (unlimited)
Strawberries (½ cup)
Coffee substitute, herbal tea, mineral wa-
ter, or seltzer

SNACK   Orange or kiwi (1)

*Recipe appears in recipe section.
†If selecting Breakfast II, serve the oatmeal (½ cup) or oatcake crackers (2) at lunch
or dinner, or as a snack, and eliminate 1 fruit serving at lunch or dinner.

WEEK 2 DAY 7

BREAKFAST I   Banana (½)
Puffed rice cereal (½ cup), rice cake (1),
or rice crackers (4)
Coffee substitute or herbal tea

OR

BREAKFAST II†   Banana (1)
Unsweetened apple juice (½ cup)
Coffee substitute or herbal tea

LUNCH   Fruit plate: Sliced apple (1), sliced banana
(½) and watermelon or Persian melon
cubes (¾ cup)
Mineral water or seltzer

DINNER   Broiled lamb chop (4 ounces)
Sautéed Cabbage with Onions* (1½ cups)
Baked acorn or butternut squash (1 cup)
Boiled Long-Grain Brown Rice* (½ cup)
Unsweetened applesauce (½ cup)
Coffee substitute, herbal tea, mineral wa-
ter, or seltzer

SNACK   Watermelon or Persian melon cubes (1 cup)

*Recipe appears in recipe section.
†If selecting Breakfast II, serve the puffed rice cereal (½ cup), rice cake (1), or rice
crackers (4) at lunch or dinner, or as a snack, and eliminate 1 fruit serving at lunch
or dinner.

WEEK 3 DAY 1

BREAKFAST I Blueberries (½ cup)
Boiled Buckwheat Groats or Kasha* (½ cup) with 1 tablespoon maple syrup (optional)
Fresh unsweetened grapefruit juice (1 cup)
Coffee substitute or herbal tea

OR

BREAKFAST II† Blueberries (1 cup)
Fresh unsweetened grapefruit juice (1 cup)
Coffee substitute or herbal tea

LUNCH Black-eyed peas or pinto beans with thyme (½ cup)
or Broiled scrod, haddock, or smelts (4 ounces)
Steamed vegetable plate: Carrots (1 cup), cauliflower (1 cup), and chickory or escarole (2 cups)
Tangerine or peach (1)
Mineral water or seltzer

DINNER Broiled scrod, haddock, or smelts (4 ounces)
Steamed Asparagus with Tarragon* (1 cup)
Steamed cauliflower (½ cup)
Chicory or escarole salad (unlimited)
Citrus Salad Dressing* (unlimited)
Blueberries (½ cup)
Coffee substitute, herbal tea, mineral water, or seltzer

SNACK Carrot juice (1 cup) or tangerine or peach (1)

---

*Recipe appears in recipe section.
†If selecting Breakfast II, serve the Buckwheat Groats or Kasha (½ cup) with 1 tablespoon maple syrup (optional) at lunch or dinner, or as a snack, and eliminate 1 fruit serving at lunch or dinner.

WEEK 3 DAY 2

BREAKFAST I   Mango or papaya (1)
Yeast-free 100% rye bread (1 slice), 100% rye crackers (2), or rye cereal (½ cup)
Coffee substitute or herbal tea

OR

BREAKFAST II†   Mango or papaya (1)
Unsweetened grape juice or apricot nectar (1 cup)
Coffee substitute or herbal tea

LUNCH   Spinach and feta salad: Spinach (unlimited), diced cucumber (½ cup), diced tomato (½ cup), and feta cheese (1 ounce)
Citrus Salad Dressing* (unlimited)
Yeast-free 100% rye bread (1 slice) or 100% rye crackers (2)
or
Broiled lean ground chuck patty or sliced beef (4 ounces)
Sliced tomato (½ cup)
Mineral water or seltzer

DINNER   Tomato juice (1 cup) with celery stick (1) and lime wedge
Broiled lean ground chuck patty or sliced roast veal (4 ounces)
Steamed brussels sprouts (1 cup)
Spinach salad (unlimited)
Citrus Salad Dressing* (unlimited)
Grapes (½ cup) or apricots (3)
Coffee substitute, herbal tea, mineral water, or seltzer

SNACK   Tomato juice (1 cup) with celery stick (1) and lime wedge

---

*Recipe appears in recipe section.
†If selecting Breakfast II, serve the yeast-free 100% rye bread (1 slice), 100% rye crackers (2) or rye cereal (½ cup) at lunch or dinner, or as a snack, and eliminate 1 fruit serving at lunch or dinner.

WEEK 3 DAY 3

BREAKFAST I Plums (2) or figs (3)
Boiled Pearl Barley* (½ cup)
Fresh unsweetened orange juice (1 cup)
Coffee substitute or herbal tea

OR
BREAKFAST II† Plums (4) or figs (6)
Fresh unsweetened orange juice (1 cup)
Coffee substitute or herbal tea

LUNCH Tuna (3½-ounce can, water packed, or 4
ounces fresh broiled)
or Broiled chicken (4 ounces)
Steamed green beans or yellow wax beans
(1 cup)
Steamed yellow squash (½ cup)
Watercress salad (unlimited)
Citrus Salad Dressing* (unlimited)
Orange (1)
Mineral water or seltzer

DINNER Chicken Satés* (4 ounces)
Stir-Fried Snow Peas with Water Chest-
nuts* (1⅛ cups)
Sautéed sliced zucchini or yellow squash
in 1 tablespoon dairy-free, low-fat marga-
rine (½ cup)
Watercress salad (unlimited)
Citrus Salad Dressing* (unlimited)
Figs (2)
Coffee substitute, herbal tea, mineral wa-
ter, or seltzer

SNACK Plums (2)

*Recipe appears in recipe section.
†If selecting Breakfast II, serve the Boiled Pearl Barley (½ cup) at lunch or dinner,
or as a snack, and eliminate 1 fruit serving at lunch or dinner.

WEEK 3 DAY 4

BREAKFAST I   Unsweetened pineapple (½ cup)
Puffed rice cereal (½ cup), rice cake (1),
or rice crackers (4)
Coffee substitute or herbal tea

OR
BREAKFAST II†   Unsweetened pineapple (1 cup)
Blackberry or black cherry juice (1 cup)
Coffee substitute or herbal tea

LUNCH   White Bean Salad* (1¼ cups) or Sliced
roast turkey (4 ounces)
Rice cake (1) or rice crackers (4)
Mineral water or seltzer

DINNER   Sliced roast turkey (4 ounces)
Steamed broccoli (1 cup)
Bibb or Boston lettuce salad (unlimited)
Citrus Salad Dressing* (unlimited)
Boiled Long-Grain Brown Rice* (½ cup)
Pineapple Mousse Sorbet* (1 cup) or un-
sweetened pineapple (½ cup)
Coffee substitute, herbal tea, mineral wa-
ter, or seltzer

SNACK   Unsweetened pineapple cubes (½ cup)

*Recipe appears in recipe section.
†If selecting Breakfast II, serve the puffed rice cereal (½ cup), rice cake (1), or rice crackers (4) at lunch or dinner, or as a snack, and eliminate 1 fruit serving at lunch or dinner.

WEEK 3 DAY 5

BREAKFAST I   Raspberries (½ cup) or honeydew or cantaloupe melon (¼)
Oatmeal (½ cup) or oatcake crackers (2) with 1 tablespoon honey
Cranberry juice (½ cup)
Coffee substitute or herbal tea

OR

BREAKFAST II†   Raspberries (1 cup) or honeydew or cantaloupe melon (½)
Cranberry juice (½ cup)
Coffee substitute or herbal tea

LUNCH   Fruit and cheese plate: Sliced pear (1) honeydew or cantaloupe melon cubes (1 cup), raspberries (½ cup), and fresh goat cheese (1 ounce)
Oatcake crackers (2)
or
Broiled sea scallops (4 ounces)
Honeydew or cantaloupe melon cubes (1 cup)
Mineral water or seltzer

DINNER   Papillote*: Sea Scallops (4 ounces)
Steamed potatoes (1 cup) with chopped parsley (¼ cup) and 1 tablespoon dairy-free low-fat margarine
Chinese Steamed Pears* (1)
Coffee substitute, herbal tea, mineral water, or seltzer

SNACK   Honeydew or cantaloupe melon (¼)

*Recipe appears in recipe section.
†If selecting Breakfast II, serve the oatmeal (½ cup) or oatcake crackers (2) with 1 tablespoon honey at lunch or dinner, or as a snack, and eliminate 1 fruit serving at lunch or dinner.

WEEK 3 DAY 6

BREAKFAST I   Blueberries or mandarin orange sections (½ cup)

Puffed millet cereal (1 cup) or Boiled Millet* (½ cup) with 1 tablespoon maple syrup

Fresh unsweetened grapefruit juice (½ cup)

Coffee substitute or herbal tea

OR

BREAKFAST II†   Blueberries or mandarin orange sections (1 cup)

Fresh unsweetened grapefruit juice (½ cup)

Coffee substitute or herbal tea

LUNCH   Salmon (3¾-ounce can, water packed, or 4 ounces fresh broiled)

or Broiled veal chop (4 ounces)

Steamed peas (½ cup)

Radish sprout, alfalfa sprout, or endive salad (unlimited)

Citrus Salad Dressing* (unlimited)

Grapefruit (½)

Mineral water or seltzer

DINNER   Broiled veal chop (4 ounces)

Baked acorn or butternut squash (1 cup)

Steamed peas (½ cup)

Endive salad (unlimited)

Citrus Salad Dressing* (unlimited)

Grapefruit Sorbet* (1 cup)

Coffee substitute, herbal tea, mineral water, or seltzer

SNACK   Celery sticks (2)

---

*Recipe appears in recipe section.

†If selecting Breakfast II, serve the puffed millet cereal (1 cup) or Boiled Millet* (½ cup) with 1 tablespoon maple syrup (optional) at lunch or dinner, or as a snack, and eliminate 1 fruit serving at lunch or dinner.

WEEK 3 DAY 7

BREAKFAST I   Mango or papaya (½)
Yeast-free 100% rye bread (1 slice), 100% rye crackers (2), or rye cereal (½ cup)
Coffee substitute or herbal tea

OR
BREAKFAST II†   Mango or papaya (1)
Unsweetened grape juice or apricot nectar (1 cup)
Coffee substitute or herbal tea

LUNCH   Spinach and feta salad: Spinach (unlimited), sliced bermuda or red onion (unlimited), artichoke hearts (¾ cup), and feta cheese (1 ounce)
Yeast-free 100% rye bread (1 slice) or 100% rye crackers (2)
Bing cherries or grapes (½ cup)
or
Sliced roast leg of lamb or broiled lamb chop with rosemary (4 ounces)
Spinach salad (unlimited)
Citrus Salad Dressing* (unlimited)
Mineral water or seltzer

DINNER   Sliced roast leg of lamb or broiled lamb chop with rosemary (4 ounces)
Broiled Eggplant* (½)
Steamed cauliflower (½ cup)
Steamed lima beans (½ cup)
Arugula salad (unlimited)
Citrus Salad Dressing* (unlimited)
Mango or papaya (½)
Coffee substitute, herbal tea, mineral water, or seltzer

SNACK   Bing cherries or grapes (½ cup)

*Recipe appears in recipe section.
†If selecting Breakfast II, serve the yeast-free 100% rye bread (1 slice), 100% rye crackers (2) or rye cereal (½ cup) at lunch or dinner, or as a snack, and eliminate 1 fruit serving at lunch or dinner.

THE 14-DAY REINTRODUCTION PLAN

When reintroducing each of the Sinister Seven Target foods, it is suggested that you do the following:

1. Reintroduce each target food in as pure a form as possible. For example, when reintroducing wheat, try to eat pure (100 percent) wheat cereal, bread, or pasta, rather than wheat products that contain other Sinister Seven foods, such as eggs, cow's milk, and yeast or other foods that you have not eaten during the Elimination phase. This will reduce the possibility that you are reacting to a food other than wheat, for example, and mistake it for wheat sensitivity.

2. Reintroduce the target food for that day, three different times throughout the day. Keep the quantities of the target food to a reasonable minimum since you will still be following the Elimination diet menu for your other food intakes.

Week 1

Day 1 *Corn*
Recipes: Tex-Mex Bean Salad with Tostaditas
Other Serving Suggestions: popcorn, puffed corn cereal, hominy, grits, corn kernels, corn on the cob, corn oil, dairy-free, low-fat corn-oil margarine, canned/bottled fruit juices sweetened with corn syrup

Day 3 *Soy Products*
Recipes: Soybean Mayonnaise
Other Serving Suggestions: Bean curd (tofu), soy oil, dairy-free, low-fat soybean margarine

Day 5   *Cane Sugar*
    Serving Suggestions: cane sugar as a topping for
    fruit or cereals, canned/bottled fruit juice sweet-
    ened with cane sugar

Day 7   *Eggs*
    Recipe: Rye Spätzle
    Other Serving Suggestions: Hard-boiled or poached
    egg, scrambled or fried egg cooked in nonstick
    pan without fat, oil, or butter

Week 2

Day 2   *Baker's and Brewer's Yeast*
    Recipes: Mustard Vinaigrette Dressing
        Leek and Red Pepper Salad
        Chicken with Bourbon Sauce
    Other Serving Suggestions: Brewer's yeast sprin-
    kled on cereal or fruit, wine, beer, or alcohol

Day 4   *Cow's Milk*
    Recipes: Linguine with 30-Minute Fresh Tomato
        Sauce (with Cow's Milk Cheese Topping)
    Other Serving Suggestions: low-fat milk, low-fat
    yogurt, low-fat cow's milk cheese, low-fat ice
    milk

Day 6   *Wheat*
    Recipes: Vegetable Rice Salad made with Maca-
        roni
        Tabouleh Salad made with Bulgur Wheat
    Other Serving Suggestions: Cream of Wheat, puffed
    wheat cereal, yeast-free 100% wheat bread,
    100% wheat pasta, bulgur

THE MAINTENANCE PLAN
FOR MEN AND WOMEN

The beauty of the maintenance stage of this diet is its flexibility; there are no hard-and-fast rules, but rather, an underlying principle, specifically, the 4-day rotation principle discussed in Chapter Six. Adapt this to your own taste and nutritional needs.

I have provided a 7-day sample menu, tailored for the individual requirements of men and women, to give you an idea of the kind of meal planning that is both ideal and possible. For the sake of variety, you may make substitutions—one carbohydrate or one protein for another—but follow the menu for portion size and balance.

Here are some useful principles to keep in mind as you stay on the maintenance diet:

1. Make sure you eat a high amount of fiber in your diet. Fiber works to keep you healthy and to fill you up. Whole-grain breads, crackers, and cereals are high in fiber, as are raw and cooked fruits and vegetables.
2. Emphasize complex carbohydrates (foods like pasta, rice, and other grains, as well as starchy vegetables like potatoes and other root vegetables and legumes) in your diet. They are ideal sources of time-release energy that your body can use most efficiently.
3. Keep the amount of fat in your diet to an absolute minimum. One good way to do this is to reduce the amount of meat in your diet and use non-stick pans with a minimum of oil for cooking.
4. Distribute your food throughout the day, eating three small meals and two snacks.
5. Remove all visible fat from foods before cooking. Peel the skin off fish and poultry before cooking.

6. If you eat fish, reduce your intake of the fatty fishes—tuna in oil, sardines in oil, rainbow trout, and whitefish.

7. Increase the amount of grains, beans, peas, and other legumes in your diet. They are a rich and filling source of protein.

8. Avoid fried foods.

9. Reduce the fatty plant foods in your diet. These include avocadoes and peanuts, and many nuts such as almonds, cashews, and brazil nuts.

10. Limit sweets—cakes, cookies, pies, muffins, and other baked goods as well as candy and ice cream. In addition to sugar, these often contain a large amount of fat.

MAINTENANCE MENU FOR WOMEN

Week 1 Day 1

BREAKFAST   Oatcakes* (3 oatcakes) or oatmeal (½ cup)
                   or yeast-free 100% rye toast (1 slice) or
                   100% rye crackers (2)
                   Apricot nectar (1 cup)
                   Coffee substitute or herbal tea

LUNCH   Spinach and egg salad: Spinach (4 cups),
                   diced cucumber (½ cup), sliced onion
                   or scallion (unlimited), sliced radish (½
                   cup), sliced hard-boiled egg (1)
                   Citrus Salad Dressing* (unlimited)
                   100% rye toast (1 slice) or 100% rye crack-
                   ers (2)
                   Plums (2)
                   Mineral water or seltzer

DINNER   Lamb Keftah* or broiled lamb chop (6
                   ounces)
                   Baba Ganouj* (¾ cup)
                   Steamed cauliflower (1 cup)
                   Warm Garlic Dressing* (2½ tablespoons)
                   Spinach salad (unlimited)
                   Citrus Salad Dressing* (unlimited)
                   Dried figs or apricots (4)
                   Coffee substitute, herbal tea, mineral wa-
                   ter, or seltzer

SNACK   Raw cauliflower (1 cup)

                   2 servings of 4 ounces wine per week *or*
                   1 serving of 3 ounces liquor per week

---

*Recipe appears in recipe section.

Week 1 Day 2

BREAKFAST
Puffed corn cereal (1 cup), or hominy or grits (½ cup)
Pineapple or prickly pear (1 cup)
Fresh unsweetened orange or tangerine juice (1 cup)
Coffee substitute or herbal tea

LUNCH
Tex-Mex salad plate: Tex-Mex Bean Salad* (1½ cups) on a bed of iceberg or romaine lettuce (unlimited)
Tostaditas (corn chips) (1 cup)
Orange or tangerine (1)
Mineral water or seltzer

DINNER
Chilled Creamy Sunchoke Soup* (1 cup) with tostaditas (corn chips) (1 cup)
Broiled chicken (6 ounces) with Ancho Sauce* (¼ cup)
Broiled Onion* (½)
Iceberg or romaine lettuce salad (unlimited)
Tomato Juice Salad Dressing* (unlimited)
Pineapple (1 cup) with shredded, unsweetened coconut (1 tablespoon)
Coffee substitute, herbal tea, mineral water, or seltzer

SNACK
Popcorn (2 cups)
Tomato juice (1 cup) with lime wedge

*Recipe appears in recipe section.

Week 1 Day 3

BREAKFAST
: Buckwheat Pancakes with Blueberries* and honey (4 pancakes)
Fresh unsweetened grapefruit juice (1 cup)
Coffee substitute or herbal tea

LUNCH
: Steamed artichoke (1)
Broiled smelt or bass (4 ounces)
Steamed peas (1 cup)
Arugula or escarole salad (unlimited)
Citrus Salad Dressing* (unlimited)
Blueberries (1 cup)
Mineral water or seltzer

DINNER
: Broiled Beefsteak, Florentine Style* (6 ounces)
Steamed asparagus (1 cup)
Steamed potatoes with sage (1 cup)
Broiled mushrooms (½ cup)
Arugula or escarole salad (unlimited)
Citrus Salad Dressing* (unlimited)
Cheese and fruit plate: Goat cheese (1 ounce), sliced pear (1), sliced peach or nectarine (1)
Coffee substitute, herbal tea, mineral water, or seltzer

SNACK
: Fresh unsweetened grapefruit juice (1 cup)
Pear or nectarine (1)

*Recipe appears in recipe section.

Week 1 Day 4

BREAKFAST Whole-wheat toast (1 slice)
Strawberries (1 cup)
Low-fat yogurt or cottage cheese (½ cup)
Coffee substitute or herbal tea

LUNCH Broiled sole or flounder (4 ounces)
Strawberries or raspberries (½ cup)
Hard French roll (1)
Mineral water or seltzer

DINNER Broiled sole or red snapper (6 ounces)
Warm Beet Salad* (¾ cup)
Hard French roll (1)
Strawberries Cardinal* (1 cup)
Coffee substitute, herbal tea, mineral water, or seltzer

SNACK Banana (1)
Kiwi (2)

*Recipe appears in recipe section.

Week 1 Day 5

BREAKFAST   Stewed rhubarb with 1 tablespoon maple
              syrup (1 cup)
              Egg (1), poached, boiled, or scrambled in
              a nonstick pan without fat
              Cranberry juice (1 cup)
              Coffee substitute or herbal tea

LUNCH   Sliced roast turkey (4 ounces)
              Baked potato (1 small)
              Coleslaw with vinaigrette dressing (1 cup)
              Unsweetened applesauce (1 cup) with rai-
              sins (¼ cup)
              Mineral water or seltzer

DINNER   Turkey Hash* (1¼ cups)
              Sautéed sugar snap peas (1 cup) or steamed
              green beans (1 cup) with 1 tablespoon
              melted dairy-free, low-fat margarine
              Baked acorn or butternut squash (½)
              Spinach salad (unlimited)
              Citrus Salad Dressing* (unlimited)
              Baked Apple* with maple syrup (1)
              Coffee substitute, herbal tea, mineral wa-
              ter, or seltzer

SNACK   Sunflower seeds (¼ cup)
              Raisins (¼ cup)
              Apple cider or juice (1 cup)

*Recipe appears in recipe section.

Week 1 Day 6

BREAKFAST   Puffed rice cereal (1 cup) or rice cakes (2)
             or rice crackers (8)
             Honeydew or cantaloupe melon (¼)
             Fresh unsweetened orange juice (1 cup)
             Coffee substitute or herbal tea

LUNCH   Tuna (3½-ounce can, water packed, or 4
             ounces fresh broiled)
             Tabouleh Salad* (1¼ cups)
             Watercress salad (unlimited)
             Citrus Salad Dressing* (unlimited)
             Plums (2) or figs (3)
             Mineral water or seltzer

DINNER   Baked Shrimp and Feta with Fresh Basil
             and Tomatoes* (1¼ cups)
             Steamed broccoli (1 cup)
             Boiled Pearl Barley* (½ cup)
             Watercress salad (unlimited)
             Tomato Juice Salad dressing* (unlimited)
             Honeydew or cantaloupe melon cubes (2
             cups)
             Coffee substitute, herbal tea, mineral wa-
             ter, or seltzer

SNACK   Tomato juice (1 cup)
             Plums (2) or figs (2)

*Recipe appears in recipe section.

Week 1 Day 7

BREAKFAST   Puffed millet cereal (1 cup) or Boiled Mil-
               let* (½ cup)
               Mandarin orange sections (1 cup) with 1
               tablespoon honey
               Unsweetened pineapple juice (1 cup)
               Coffee substitute or herbal tea

LUNCH   Steamed vegetable platter: Snow peas (1
               cup), bok choy or Chinese cabbage (2
               cups) and carrots (1 cup) garnished with
               herbs
               Lychees (1 cup) and loquats (1 cup)
               Mineral water or seltzer

DINNER   Chinese Lettuce Packages* (2 cups)
               Stir-Fried Snow Peas with Water Chest-
               nuts* (1⅛ cups)
               Bean sprouts (1 cup)
               Fruit platter: Mandarin orange sections (½
               cup), lychees (½ cup), and loquats (½
               cup)
               Coffee substitute, herbal tea, mineral wa-
               ter, or seltzer

SNACK   Unsweetened pineapple juice (1 cup)
               Carrot sticks (1 cup)

*Recipe appears in recipe section.

MAINTENANCE MENU FOR MEN

Week 1 Day 1

BREAKFAST
Oatcakes* (3 oatcakes) or oatmeal (½ cup) or yeast-free 100% rye toast (1 slice) or 100% rye crackers (2)
Apricot nectar (1 cup)
Coffee substitute or herbal tea

LUNCH
Broiled halibut or swordfish (4 ounces)
Spinach and egg salad: Spinach (4 cups), diced cucumber (½ cup), sliced onion or scallion (unlimited), sliced radish (½ cup), sliced hard-boiled egg (1)
Citrus Salad Dressing* (unlimited)
100% rye toast (2 slices) or 100% rye crackers (4)
Mineral water or seltzer

DINNER
Lamb Keftah* or broiled lamb chop (6 ounces)
Baba Ganouj* (¾ cup)
Steamed cauliflower (1 cup)
Warm Garlic Dressing* (2½ tablespoons)
Spinach salad (unlimited)
Citrus Salad Dressing* (unlimited)
Dried figs or apricots (4)
Coffee substitute, herbal tea, mineral water, or seltzer

SNACK
Raw cauliflower (1 cup)
Plum (1)
Hard-boiled egg (1)

*Recipe appears in recipe section.

Week 1 Day 2

BREAKFAST   Puffed corn cereal (1 cup), or hominy or
grits (½ cup)
Pineapple or prickly pear (1 cup)
Fresh unsweetened orange or tangerine juice
(1 cup)
Coffee substitute or herbal tea

LUNCH   Broiled chicken (4 ounces)
Tex-Mex salad plate: Tex-Mex Bean Salad*
(1½ cups) on a bed of iceberg or romaine
lettuce (unlimited)
Tostaditas (corn chips) (1 cup)
Orange or tangerine (2)
Mineral water or seltzer

DINNER   Chilled Creamy Sunchoke Soup* (1 cup)
Broiled chicken (8 ounces) with Ancho
Sauce* (½ cup)
Broiled Onion* (1)
Iceberg or romaine lettuce salad (unlimited)
Tomato Juice Salad Dressing* (unlimited)
Pineapple (1 cup) with shredded, unsweet-
ened coconut (2 tablespoons)
Coffee substitute, herbal tea, mineral wa-
ter, or seltzer

SNACK   Popcorn (2 cups)
Tomato juice (1 cup) with lime wedge

*Recipe appears in recipe section.

Week 1 Day 3

BREAKFAST   Buckwheat Pancakes with Blueberries* and honey (4 pancakes)
Fresh unsweetened grapefruit juice (1 cup)
Coffee substitute or herbal tea

LUNCH   Steamed artichoke (1)
Broiled smelt or bass (4 ounces)
Steamed peas (1 cup)
Arugula or escarole salad (unlimited)
Citrus Salad Dressing* (unlimited)
Blueberries (1 cup)
Mineral water or seltzer

DINNER   Broiled Beefsteak, Florentine Style* (8 ounces)
Steamed asparagus (1 cup)
Steamed potatoes with sage (1 cup)
Broiled mushrooms (1 cup)
Arugula or escarole salad (unlimited)
Citrus Salad Dressing* (unlimited)
Cheese and fruit plate: Goat cheese (2 ounces), sliced pear (1), sliced peach or nectarine (1)
Coffee substitute, herbal tea, mineral water, or seltzer

SNACK   Fresh unsweetened grapefruit juice (2 cups)
Pear or nectarine (2)

*Recipe appears in recipe section.

Week 1 Day 4

BREAKFAST   Whole-wheat toast (2 slices)
Strawberries (1 cup)
Low-fat yogurt or cottage cheese (1 cup)
Coffee substitute or herbal tea

LUNCH   Broiled sole or flounder (4 ounces)
Strawberries or raspberries (1 cup)
Hard French roll (1)
Mineral water or seltzer

DINNER   Broiled sole or red snapper (8 ounces)
Warm Beet Salad* (¾ cup)
Hard French roll (1)
Strawberries Cardinal* (1 cup)
Coffee substitute, herbal tea, mineral water,
    or seltzer

SNACK   Banana (2)
Kiwi (3)

*Recipe appears in recipe section.

Week 1 Day 5

BREAKFAST   Stewed rhubarb with 1 tablespoon maple
       syrup (1 cup)
      Eggs (2), poached, boiled, or scrambled in
       a nonstick pan without fat
      Cranberry juice (1 cup)
      Coffee substitute or herbal tea

LUNCH   Sliced roast turkey (6 ounces)
      Baked potato (1 medium)
      Coleslaw with vinaigrette dressing (1 cup)
      Unsweetened applesauce (1 cup) with rai-
       sins (¼ cup)
      Mineral water or seltzer

DINNER   Turkey Hash* (1¼ cups)
      Sautéed sugar snap peas (1 cup) or steamed
       green beans (1 cup) with 1 tablespoon
       melted dairy-free, low-fat margarine
      Baked acorn or butternut squash (½)
      Spinach salad (unlimited)
      Citrus Salad Dressing* (unlimited)
      Baked Apple* with maple syrup (1)
      Coffee substitute, herbal tea, mineral wa-
       ter, or seltzer

SNACK   Sunflower seeds (¼ cup)
      Raisins (½ cup)
      Apple cider or juice (1 cup)

*Recipe appears in recipe section.

Week 1 Day 6

BREAKFAST   Puffed rice cereal (1 cup) or rice cakes (2)
               or rice crackers (8)
               Honeydew or cantaloupe melon (½)
               Fresh unsweetened orange juice (1 cup)
               Coffee substitute or herbal tea

LUNCH   Tuna (6½-ounce can, water packed, or 6
               ounces fresh broiled)
               Tabouleh Salad* (1¼ cups)
               Watercress salad (unlimited)
               Citrus Salad Dressing* (unlimited)
               Plums (2) or figs (3)
               Mineral water or seltzer

DINNER   Baked Shrimp and Feta with Fresh Basil
               and Tomatoes* (1¼ cups)
               Steamed broccoli (1 cup)
               Boiled Pearl Barley* (1 cup)
               Watercress salad (unlimited)
               Tomato Juice Salad Dressing* (unlimited)
               Honeydew or cantaloupe melon cubes (2
               cups)
               Coffee substitute, herbal tea, mineral wa-
               ter, or seltzer

SNACK   Tomato juice (1 cup)
               Plums (3) or figs (3)
               Feta cheese (2 ounces)

*Recipe appears in recipe section.

Week 1 Day 7

BREAKFAST   Puffed millet cereal (1 cup) or Boiled Mil-
let* (½ cup)
Mandarin orange sections (1 cup) with 1
tablespoon honey
Unsweetened pineapple juice (1 cup)
Coffee substitute or herbal tea

LUNCH   Broiled bluefish or swordfish (4 ounces)
Steamed vegetable platter: Snow peas (1
cup), bok choy or Chinese cabbage (2
cups) and carrots (1 cup) garnished with
herbs
Lychees (1 cup) and loquats (1 cup)
Mineral water or seltzer

DINNER   Chinese Lettuce Packages* (2 cups)
Stir-Fried Snow Peas with Water Chestnuts* (1⅛ cups)
Bean sprouts (2 cups)
Fruit platter: Mandarin orange sections (½
cup), lychees (½ cup), and loquats (½
cup)
Coffee substitute, herbal tea, mineral water, or seltzer

SNACK   Unsweetened pineapple juice (1 cup)
Carrot sticks (1 cup)
Pears (2)

*Recipe appears in recipe section.

IMMUNE POWER DIET TIPS

Of course the ideal way to follow the Immune Power Diet is to eat at home through the entire period so that you have absolute control over your food. Well, this is not an ideal world. Few of us can avoid travel and having to eat in restaurants—certainly not my patients with their high-power careers. So here are a few tips to help maximize Immune Power nutrition when your daily routine is unavoidably disturbed.

EATING OUT—HEALTHILY

Restaurants are the downfall of many dieters, but they don't have to be. You can find appropriate foods at virtually any kind of restaurant, from a hash-house to a four-star dining room. All you need to do is carefully inspect the menu.

- Get out of your rut. Here's your chance to try new and different dishes. Don't automatically order the same old thing; take a moment to study the options before you.
- Don't always eat every course on the menu. Try something different. Drop the main course. Build your meal just from appetizers, or appetizers and salads. Be creative.
- In order to keep the four-day rotation and the principles of sound immune dieting, some patients like to bring along the list of what they ate during the last three days to make sure they don't repeat.
- Many restaurants have dieter's plates of tuna, hamburger patty, sliced, roasted meat, fresh fruit, and salad bars. For dessert, concentrate on fresh fruit.

- If you are in the Elimination diet phase, concentrate on simply prepared main dishes: broiled or steamed meats, fish, poultry, or vegetables.
- Uncertain just what the restaurant will have? By all means take along your own food items. For example, one patient always brings along a little bag of the herbal tea for that day, and just orders hot water as a beverage.
- The first terrible temptation of any meal eaten out comes when the bread basket arrives on the table. Remember, those breads, crackers, and snacks are chock full of many of the Sinister Seven Target foods— eggs, wheat, cow's milk, and yeast. If you are alone, have the basket of bread removed. If there are others, bring along your own rice crackers, oat cake crackers, or rye crackers. That way, you can eat along with your companions while avoiding your danger foods.
- Avoiding yeast means avoiding alcohol. When everybody else orders a cocktail, order a drink like a Virgin Mary (*without* Worcestershire Sauce), natural fruit juices, or mineral water with a wedge of lime, lemon, or orange.

TRAVEL IS SO . . . SLIMMING

The old saying tells us that "travel is broadening," but it doesn't have to be—at least, not for your waistline. There are several ways to stick to the principles of the Immune Power Diet when you are en route.

- Most airlines offer a wide variety of meals that you can special order, a service which few people know about. They often have recommended foods such as mixed seafood platter, fresh fruit plate, or a "dietetic'' hamburger meal. Ask about these when you make your reservation.

- Often, flying is exactly the best time *not* to eat, or to eat very lightly. Long plane rides can drain your energy and disturb your body clock. You'll feel better if you steer clear of heavy meals.

- Try packing a light snack or meal based on one of the daily Immune Power menus. You will eat better, and should arrive feeling more rested and energetic.

- Be extra sure to drink plenty of non-alcoholic beverages when you fly. Dehydration is in a large part responsible for jet lag, so take in plenty of fluids.

MAKING POSITIVE IMMUNE NUTRITION A FAMILY AFFAIR

Like many of my patients, you probably share household meals with your spouse, family, or lover. Eating with others, and preparing food for them, can make it harder to get on and stay on any diet program, especially if your nearest and dearest isn't satisfied by the kind, variety, or quantity of food specified in the diet. Because so many of my patients find themselves in this situation, here are a few suggestions I have found make it extra easy to bring the Immune Power Diet into your family.

- *Fresh raw fruit* is an important part of the desserts and snacks on your diet. Obviously, there's no reason your family can't enjoy those same fruits. But if some sweet tooths aren't satisfied by raw fruit, let them dress it up a bit—put their portions over ice cream, sherbet, or sorbet.

- Many kinds of *fresh vegetables* are called for in the Immune Power Diet. You will usually want to steam them, and eat them plain. For the family, though, there are a variety of quick and easy toppings and sauces to improve the vegetables. For example, they may want them topped with herb butter. That makes cooking and serving a breeze—serve everyone the same thing, then put the topping on the table for those who want to help themselves.

- *Meat* is the biggest area where the whole family will benefit most from the Immune Power Diet. Most Americans eat far too much fatty meat; the broiled lean meat called for in the diet will be good for the whole family.

- *Increase quantities* for other family members. The quantity of food counts as much as the nutrient balance in the Immune Power Diet. That means, when your diet plan calls for four ounces of chicken breast, for example, there's no reason not to give larger helpings to others. They'll stay satisfied, and you'll not only save work, but lose weight!

- *Make the diet a family project*. Most people are surprised at how positive the diet can be for the whole family. And why not—after all, here's the chance for everybody to be healthier, happier, slimmer, and more energetic. It will give you something important to share and to talk about at the table. Like so many projects, it's easier, and more fun, when everybody joins in.

THE RECIPES: SAY GOODBYE TO "CAVEMAN CUISINE"

Variety is not only the spice of life, it's absolutely essential for healthy eaters. Too many diet plans rely on what I call "caveman cuisine." They are based on the same primitive eating principles our ancestors used in their caves millions of years ago: a too-meager selection of oft-repeated rudimentary foods.

Such caveman cuisine is not only unappetizing, it is downright unhealthy. The recipes in this book include a wide range of ingredients and styles of preparation. Most people on the diet find that they are eating—and enjoying—a wider variety of food than ever before.

The recipes range from very simple dishes to fine gourmet treats and include many ethnic and regional cuisines: Middle Eastern, Greek, French, Italian, Chinese, and American Regional. They are organized into main food categories: broths and soups, breakfast foods, appetizers, vegetable salads, legume and grain salads, vegetable dishes, grain dishes, dressings and sauces, main dishes, and desserts.

Many are classics which have traditionally contained one or more of the Sinister Seven foods. Now you can enjoy favorites like pancakes, "breaded" foods, and salad dressings in versions which omit most of those forbidden ingredients, substituting non-allergenic foods. You may have discovered in the detoxification diet that you're allergic or sensitive to some particular food item included in this diet. In that case, common sense prevails: Don't include it in the recipe; substitute something you *can* have.

All of the recipes follow the best nutritional principles: high fiber, low sodium, low fats, and a balanced protein to carbohydrate ratio. In addition, these recipes eliminate "empty calorie" foods.

Many of the simpler, "no-fuss" recipes are used in the 21-day Elimination phase of the diet. The more special gourmet dishes are reserved for the time when you can branch out and experiment on your own in the maintenance phase, but throughout the diet your meals will be delicious as well as health-building.

Before you begin to read about the adventures in good eating you'll find in the Immune Power recipes, I want to tell you about a very special patient. Mary Beth, a petite brown-haired blue-eyed young woman, came to my office with a host of minor problems—aching arms and shoulders, swelling hands, tension, insomnia, a few extra pounds that wouldn't go away—that added up to a major drain on the energy necessary to be both a housewife and a professional woman. "I've had one cold after another for the past two years," she told me, "and I seem to get the flu every other month. Nothing seems to help."

After testing Mary Beth, I discovered that she had severe sensitivities to six of the Sinister Seven foods and less important reactions to others. As a trained home economist, Mary Beth not only made the Immune Power Diet work for her, she has used her expertise to devise these delicious recipes that will work for you! Incidentally, Mary Beth's husband is also on the Immune Power Diet, which has not only enabled him to lose fifteen pounds but cleared up his lifelong, severe asthma.

As you use the Immune Power recipes, remember that they are all triple-tested, in the home by a professional cook, in a cooking school, and by my patients who attend Mary Beth's seminars on putting Immune Power into your own kitchen.

Enjoy!

SHOPPING TIPS

The Immune Power Diet recipes call for common, easily available foods that, for the most part, can be purchased at your local grocery store. Here are some tips to make shopping easier:

- Your nearest health food store is also a very good place to shop. There you should be able to find a large selection of grains, broths without MSG or yeast, yeast-free bread, dairy-free margarine and products sweetened with honey or pure maple syrup.

- Specialty food stores usually carry a selection of oils, special pastas, spices, and other special ingredients that you may want to use in your recipes. They are often a good place to buy that "special something" that will give your diet originality.

- Read all ingredient labels. You will be amazed at how many of the Sinister Seven ingredients repeatedly find their way into food products called "natural." This is true not just for Sinister Seven foods, but for a whole range of food preservatives, stabilizers, emulsifiers, flavorings, humectants, and other food additives. Read carefully before you buy.

- Keep your menu fresh and seasonal. Avoid frozen, canned, processed, or bottled products whenever possible. This allows you to buy foods that not only taste good, but still retain their nutritional value.

- Buy in small quantities. Again, this protects the vitamin and mineral value of your foods by reducing storage time. If you must buy in larger quantities, divide the food into single serving portions, wrap it well, and freeze it. Thaw overnight in your refrigerator before preparation.

- Remember that when you buy raw fish, meat, or poultry, the raw weight will always be greater than cooked weight. So always buy a little extra because you will lose a substantial portion of these foods when they are trimmed or boned.

   This also holds true for grains and cereals. When the Elimination diet specifies a certain amount of food, it means cooked, not raw, amount.

WHEN YOU'RE THIRSTY . . .

What we drink has a large effect on how satisfied we feel, so you should be aware of all the drinks allowable on the diet.

- Coffee substitutes, found in health food stores or specialty food shops, taste almost exactly like coffee. Since they are made from grains, spices, and dried fruits, they contain no harmful caffeine.
- Mineral water is not only popular, it's wonderfully healthy for you. If you choose seltzer water, make sure it has no sodium added.
- Fruit juices are included in the diet menus. On the days you eat cereal in the morning, but can't have milk, moisten the cereal with the natural fruit juice recommended for that day. Remember, drink only natural, unsweetened juices.

COOKING TIPS

- Do not use vegetable cooking sprays. They often contain soy-bean products and alcohol, so they can be hidden sources of the Sinister Seven. These preparations, and the propellants they use, can *create* food sensitivities.
- Trim all the visible fat off of your meat, fish, and poultry before cooking. Remove chicken and turkey skin before cooking.
- Use broth for sautéeing and stir frying, rather than butter, margarine, or oils.
- Use low-fat dairy products when possible.
- Rely on the natural sodium content of ingredients for flavor. With very few exceptions, these recipes contain no added sodium.

COOKING EQUIPMENT

If you become a serious Immune Power cook, you may eventually want to add these items to your kitchen.

- A steamer for vegetables. Steamers run from simple, fold-out metal frames to complex units with built-in heating. Any kind of steamer will help preserve the vital nutrients in the cooked food.
- A nonstick pan. I recommend a heavy pan such as the DuPont Silverstone®. By cooking with a nonstick pan, you need less oil, butter, or margarine in some recipes.
- A Römertopf® clay casserole. These special, sealed casseroles virtually eliminate the need to add any kind of cooking oil.

BROILING MEATS, POULTRY, FISH, AND VEGETABLES

Broiling is a fast and efficient way to cook many ingredients without adding any butter, margarine, or oil.

Preparing the Ingredients for Broiling: Rinse under cold running water to wash, if necessary, and pat dry. Remove the skin to substantially reduce fat content.

How to Broil: Place the broiler pan 4 inches from the heat source and preheat the broiler. Rub the ingredients with sliced garlic, citrus juice, onion juice, and/or herbs if desired; remember not to repeat any of these flavorings more than once every four days. Arrange the ingredients on the pan in a single layer. Broil to desired doneness, turning once.

Remember that the weight of meat, poultry, and fish

listed in the menu plans is *cooked* weight. When purchasing these ingredients, allow for the additional weight of refuse (bone, skin, fat, gristle) and the loss of a small quantity of water, juice, and rendered fat. Therefore, purchase 1 to 3 ounces more than the final cooked weight. Since ingredients vary with season and maturity, the following broiling time for rare, medium, or well-done cooking is approximate: 4 minutes for rare to 10 minutes for well done, for ¾-inch thickness.

STEAMING VEGETABLES AND FISH

Steaming is the most nutritious and fastest way to cook vegetables and fish. If you do not have a steamer and are interested in purchasing one, you can select from the following excellent products: a collapsible and expanding stainless-steel steamer, available in most department, hardware, and variety stores, or a metal or bamboo steamer, available in department and specialty kitchen-ware stores.

The collapsible stainless-steel steamer can hold up to four portions of vegetables or fish filets and must be put inside a deep pot with a cover.

The metal or bamboo steamers are self-contained units and need no additional equipment. I highly recommend either of these because they are versatile enough to hold amounts from a single portion of vegetables or fish to several ears of corn or a whole fish.

Preparing the Vegetables for Steaming: Wash the vegetables well in cold water and drain. Cut the firm vegetables like potatoes, turnips, carrots, parsnips, rutabaga, winter squash, and zucchini and other squash into 2-inch pieces for faster steaming. Separate broccoli and cauliflower into small flowerets. The tiny vegetables like corn kernels, lima beans, and peas may be put into heatproof bowls.

Semihard vegetables like asparagus and green beans may be left whole. Leafy greens such as cabbage, spinach, bok choy, and chickory may be thickly sliced or left whole with the leaves separated.

Preparing the Fish for Steaming: Rinse the fish well under cold running water, drain, and pat dry. Place it on foil or a heatproof plate.

How to Steam: Fill the pot or steamer with water. If using the collapsible stainless-steel steamer, make sure that the water does not touch the bottom of the steamer. Bring the water to a boil and add the ingredients. Steam the ingredients until tender; that is, when easily pierced in the center with a fork or the sharp point of a knife. Remove immediately. Either puree at this point or leave whole. Sprinkle with herbs, if desired, remembering not to repeat them more than once every four days. Serve hot, or cool and chill for serving in a cold dish at a later time.

The following steaming times are approximate, since ingredients vary with season and maturity: firm vegetables, 10 to 20 minutes; broccoli and cauliflower flowerets, 8 to 10 minutes; zucchini and summer squash, 4 to 6 minutes; corn kernels, lima beans, and peas, 5 to 10 minutes; semihard vegetables, 4 to 10 minutes; leafy greens, 2 to 10 minutes; whole fish, 10 to 15 minutes per 1-inch thickness; fish fillet, 4 to 5 minutes per ½-inch thickness.

Garnish: Sprinkle fresh and dried herbs, such as chives, parsley, or sage, over steamed fish or vegetables.

NOTE: The recipes have been coded E, R, or M (or a combination) to indicate whether they fit into the Elimination, Reintroduction, or Maintenance stages of the diet. The quantities called for in the diet menus are for 1 serving. If following a recipe that yields more than 1 serving, simply divide its quantity by the number it yields to prepare 1 serving.

Broths and Soups

All of the recipes in the Broth and Soup section are cow's milk-free, cane sugar-free, egg-free, corn-free, and wheat-free. All of the recipes are also soy-free and baker's and brewer's yeast-free except for the Vegetable Broth.

Most of the commercial canned broths available for purchase today contain monosodium glutamate (MSG), salt, yeast, and other additives. Therefore, it is best if you make your own broths so you can control the ingredients you ingest. I recommend that you make pure broths, especially for the Elimination diet, without extra vegetables, herbs, and spices, as it is easier to repeat only that one ingredient once every four days rather than all the ingredients that usually make up a broth. The following recipes show how to prepare delicious broths easily. Remember to use the chicken broth on the day you eat chicken, beef broth on the day you eat beef or veal, etc., so that you have two forms of the same ingredient on the same day.

Chicken Broth E, R, M

Yield: 4 cups

3 pounds chicken, chopped   8 cups cold water
into 2-inch pieces

1. Arrange the chicken in a single layer, if possible, in
   the bottom of a stockpot. Pour in the cold water.
2. Over medium heat, bring the water to a boil and continue to boil for 5 minutes. Skim off any scum that
   floats on the surface. Reduce the heat to low and
   simmer for 2 to 3 hours. Check occasionally to make
   sure the chicken is not sticking to the pot and burning.
   (The water should *never* boil after the initial 5 minutes;
   if it does and reduces too quickly, the essential oils
   which provide most of the flavor will evaporate. The
   result will be a broth rich in gelatin with very little
   flavor.)
3. After simmering for 2 to 3 hours, taste the chicken. If
   the chicken has no flavor of its own, the broth is done.
   If the chicken has some flavor, simmer until all of its
   flavor has been extracted into the broth, but not more
   than 1 hour more.
4. When the broth is finished, remove the chicken. Strain
   the broth through cheesecloth or a fine-mesh colander.
   Cool before refrigerating or the broth will turn sour.
   Cover tightly and refrigerate overnight so any fat can
   rise to the surface and harden. Remove the fat. Continue to refrigerate up to 5 days or freeze up to 2
   months.

VARIATION: A bouquet garni may be added to the broth after the initial 5 minutes of boiling and subsequent skimming of the surface. Select any or all of the following and wrap in cheesecloth: 1 leek, white part only, split and cleaned, or 1 small peeled whole onion; 1 large carrot cut into 2-inch sections; 1 stalk celery cut into 2-inch sections; 1 whole dried bay leaf; 2 sprigs fresh thyme or ½ teaspoon dried; and/or 6 parsley stems.

Turkey Broth E, R, M

Yield: 4 cups

**3 pounds turkey, chopped   8 cups cold water
   into 2-inch pieces**

1. Arrange the turkey in a single layer, if possible, in the bottom of a stockpot. Pour in the cold water.
2. Over medium heat, bring the water to a boil and continue to boil for 5 minutes. Skim off any scum that floats on the surface. Reduce heat to low and simmer for 2 to 3 hours. Check occasionally to make sure the turkey is not sticking to the pot and burning. (The water should *never* boil after the initial 5 minutes; if it does and reduces too quickly, the essential oils which provide most of the flavor will evaporate. The result will be a broth rich in gelatin with very little flavor.)
3. After simmering for 2 to 3 hours, taste the turkey. If the turkey has no flavor of its own, the broth is done. If the turkey has some flavor, simmer until all of its flavor has been extracted into the broth, but not more than 1 hour more.
4. When the broth is finished, remove the turkey. Strain the broth through cheesecloth or a fine-mesh colander. Cool before refrigerating or the broth will turn sour. Cover tightly and refrigerate overnight so any fat can rise to the surface and harden. Remove the fat. Continue to refrigerate up to 5 days or freeze up to 2 months.

VARIATION: A bouquet garni may be added to the broth after the initial 5 minutes of boiling and subsequent skimming of the surface. Select any or all of the following and wrap in cheesecloth: 1 leek, white part only, split and cleaned, or 1 small peeled whole onion; 1 large carrot cut into 2-inch sections; 1 stalk celery cut into 2-inch sections; 1 whole dried bay leaf; 2 sprigs fresh thyme or ½ teaspoon dried; and/or 6 parsley stems.

Chilled Creamy Sunchoke Soup M

Yield: 4 servings

Sunchokes, or Jerusalem artichokes, are a greatly under-utilized starchy vegetable that contain virtually no fat, but do contain Vitamins A and C, phosphorus, calcium, magnesium, and iron. They make a luscious, creamy soup similar to vichyssoise, or chilled cream of potato and leek soup, without adding a trace of cream or potato. Easy to make, this soup may be prepared a few days in advance of serving, making it ideal for entertaining.

*1 pound sunchokes
(Jerusalem artichokes),
   peeled and cut into
   1-inch pieces
1¼ cups broth (chicken,*

*turkey, or vegetable),
   divided
¾ cup (2 small) sliced
   leeks, stalk only*

Garnish

*2 teaspoons fresh
   snipped chives (optional)*

*Freshly ground white
   pepper and allspice to
   taste*

1. Steam the sunchokes until tender, about 10 minutes. Meanwhile, put the broth into a saucepan, add the leeks, and simmer until the leeks are tender, about 10 minutes.
2. Place the sunchokes in a food processor or blender and puree. Remove the leeks from the broth with a slotted spoon; add them to the sunchokes and puree. Slowly pour in 1 cup broth while pureeing. (Add the additional ¼ cup broth if desired.) Season to taste.

3. For fullest flavor, prepare one day in advance and chill tightly covered. Serve slightly chilled with the garnish sprinkled on top if desired.

Beef Broth E, R, M

Yield: 4 cups

*3 pounds chuck, chopped   1 pound beef bones, split
   into 2-inch pieces   8 cups cold water*

1. Arrange the meat and bones in a single layer, if possible, in the bottom of a stockpot. Pour in the cold water.
2. Over medium heat, bring the water to a boil and continue to boil for 5 minutes. Skim off any scum that floats on the surface. Reduce the heat to low and simmer for 2 to 3 hours. Check occasionally to make sure the meat is not sticking to the pot and burning. (The water should *never* boil after the initial 5 minutes; if it does and reduces too quickly, the essential oils which provide most of the flavor will evaporate. The result will be a broth rich in gelatin with very little flavor.)
3. After simmering for 2 to 3 hours, taste the meat. If the meat has no flavor of its own, the broth is done. If the meat has some flavor, simmer until all of its flavor has been extracted into the broth, but not more than 1 hour more.
4. When the broth is finished, remove the meat and bones. strain the broth through cheesecloth or a fine-mesh colander. Cool before refrigerating or the broth will turn sour. Cover tightly and refrigerate overnight so any fat can rise to the surface and harden. Remove the fat. Continue to refrigerate up to 5 days or freeze up to 2 months.

VARIATIONS: 1. For veal broth, use 3 pounds veal bones, split, with 1 pound stewing veal.

2. A bouquet garni may be added to the broth after the initial 5 minutes of boiling and subsequent skimming of the surface. Select any or all of the following and wrap in cheesecloth: 1 leek, white part only, split and cleaned, or 1 small peeled whole onion; 1 large carrot cut into 2-inch sections; 1 stalk celery cut into 2-inch sections; 1 whole dried bay leaf; 2 sprigs fresh thyme or ½ teaspoon dried; and/or 6 parsley stems.

Vegetable Broth M

Yield: 4 cups

This is a delicious, satisfying broth that can be substituted for any kind of meat or poultry broth.

*1 small pad (4 ounces)
   spicy or plain bean
   curd (tofu)
½ cup chopped celery
¾ cup chopped carrot
½ small yellow onion*

*12 dried Chinese black
   mushrooms or 12
   sliced fresh mushrooms
4½ cups cold water*

Combine all ingredients in a saucepan. Bring the water to a boil, reduce to a simmer, and cook for 45 minutes. Strain. Refrigerate up to 5 days or freeze up to 2 months.

Parsnip and Leek Soup E, R, M

Yield: 4 servings

This delicious vegetable soup is rich and creamy and very simple to prepare. It makes a satisfying main course as well as a first course and can be served warmed or chilled. Parsnip and Leek Soup is best if prepared one day in advanced of serving, and it can be successfully frozen for up to one month.

1 pound (3 medium) parsnips, peeled and quartered
2½–3 cups broth (vegetable, chicken, or veal), divided
½ cup (1 small) sliced leek, stalk only, or onion

⅛ cup diced carrot or celery
Freshly ground white pepper, nutmeg, and allspice to taste

Garnish (optional)

1 teaspoon ground coriander

1 teaspoon ground cardamom

1. Steam parsnips until tender when pierced with a fork in the center, about 10 to 12 minutes.
2. In 2½ cups broth, simmer the leek or onion and carrot or celery until tender, about 20 minutes.
3. Place the parsnips, leek or onion, and carrot or celery in a food processor or blender and puree until smooth. Pour in the broth and puree again. (Add the additional ½ cup broth if desired.) Season to taste.

4. For fullest flavor, prepare one day in advance and chill tightly covered. Serve either slightly chilled or warmed— avoid extreme temperatures. If desired, sprinkle garnish on top before serving.

VARIATION: *Rutabaga and Leek Soup* is equally delicious. For this version, simply substitute 1 pound rutabaga (1 small) for the parsnips and increase the broth to 3½ to 4 cups. Garnish with 1 teaspoon ground coriander or mace.

Breakfast Foods

All of the recipes in this section are corn-free, soy-free, cane sugar-free, wheat-free, baker's and brewer's yeast-free, egg-free and cow's milk-free.

Oatcakes M

Yield: 2 servings

If you like oats, you'll love this traditional Irish breakfast—
the essence of oats, creamy inside and golden toasted
outside and a good source of fiber. For a country treat,
serve them with warmed maple syrup.

1 cup rolled oats
  ⅛ teaspoon baking soda
  2½ tablespoons dairy-
free low-fat marga-
  rine, divided
  ¼ cup boiling water

Garnish (optional)

⅓ cup maple syrup, warmed
  or ¼ cup honey

1. In a blender or food processor (use the steel chopping blade), chop the oats to a coarse meal. Transfer to a mixing bowl and add the baking soda.
2. Melt 2 tablespoons margarine, pour into the oatmeal
   and mix well. Slowly pour in the boiling water, stirring
   constantly and scraping the sides of the bowl, until a
   sticky batter develops. Let rest for 3 minutes.
3. Meanwhile, heat a nonstick sauté pan or griddle until
   warm. Melt the remaining margarine. Drop 6 spoonfuls
   of batter onto the pan and pat down until only ¼ inch
   high. Cook over low to medium heat until crisp and
   golden brown, about 5 to 7 minutes. Turn over and
   repeat. Serve.

Buckwheat Pancakes
with Blueberries M

Yield: 4 servings

These are a comforting breakfast on a cold morning.

1 cup buckwheat flour
¾ teaspoon cream of
tartar
½ teaspoon baking soda
4 tablespoons melted

dairy-free low-fat
margarine, divided
1½ to 2 cups boiling
water

Garnish (optional)
¾ cup fresh blueberries
⅓ cup honey, preferably
buckwheat or tupelo

1. Sift flour, cream of tartar, and baking soda together in a large mixing bowl.
2. Melt 3 tablespoons margarine, pour into the flour, and mix well.
3. Slowly pour in 1½ cups boiling water, stirring constantly and scraping the sides of the bowl, until a smooth batter develops. Add up to the additional ½ cup boiling water if necessary. The batter should have the consistency of thick honey. If using the blueberries, stir into the batter now—or reserve and sprinkle over the cooked pancakes just before serving.
4. Heat a 12- to 14-inch nonstick sauté pan until warm and melt 1½ teaspoons margarine.
5. Using about half of the batter, pour about 3 tablespoons of batter for each pancake onto the cooking surface.

Smooth the batter out so each pancake is only ¼ inch thick (except for the height of the blueberries). Lower heat and cook the pancake for 5 to 6 minutes or until the edges turn darker and the centers develop air bubbles and puff up. The pancakes are ready to be turned over when they slide easily in the pan.

6. Turn each pancake over. Cook for 3 to 4 minutes. The pancakes are done when they spring back when tapped in the center. Transfer to a plate and keep warm in a 200° oven. Repeat with the remaining batter following Steps 4 to 6.

7. Serve with honey if desired, or top with more blueberries.

Appetizers

Both the recipes in the Appetizer section are corn-free, soy-free, cane sugar-free, egg-free, wheat-free, baker's and brewer's yeast-free, and cow's milk-free.

Feta with Herbs M

Yield: 4 servings

Fresh, creamy feta is a nonfermented sheep's milk cheese that is quite versatile. While it is often served in salads, here feta is combined with herbs to give it a special flavor. Marinated feta can be served as a dish in itself and is especially good with beef and lamb. Ideal for entertaining, this dish should be prepared in advance and will remain in perfect condition for up to 5 days.

1 teaspoon fresh thyme or   *8 ounces feta, cut into*
   ¼ teaspoon dried   *½-inch slices or*
   thyme   *broken into 1-inch*
1 teaspoon fresh   *chunks*
   oregano or ¼ tea-
   spoon dried oregano

1. Select a deep, narrow container for the cheese. Place the cheese in the container and sprinkle with herbs. (If using slices, stand them up side by side.)
2. Cover tightly and refrigerate for at least 4 hours to 1 day before serving.

Vegetable Salads

Baba Ganouj M

Yield: 2 servings

Baba Ganouj is a Middle Eastern eggplant dish that makes an excellent cold appetizer or side dish. This savory vegetable cream is low in calories, yet rich in taste.

*1 pound (1 medium)
  eggplant
⅛ teaspoon minced
  garlic
2⅓ teaspoons fresh lemon
  juice*

*1 tablespoon tahini
  paste
A generous pinch of
  cumin (optional)*

1. Trim and quarter eggplant lengthwise.
2. Broil eggplant 4 inches from heat source for 10 to 15 minutes, turning once to brown evenly. The eggplant is done when it is soft and exuding some water on its surface. Cool and peel.
3. Place the eggplant between several sheets of absorbent toweling to rid it of excess water.
4. Puree the eggplant and garlic in a blender or food processor. Add the lemon juice and tahini paste and blend until fluffy. (If using the cumin, add and blend.)
5. Chill for 2 to 24 hours before serving.

NOTE: If the tahini paste (ground raw sesame seeds) is separated, with oil floating on top, stir until emulsified or blended and then use. Store unused paste in the refrigerator for up to 2 months.

Vegetable Salads

All of the recipes in the Vegetable Salad section are corn-free, soy-free, cane sugar-free, egg-free, wheat-free, and cow's milk-free. All of the recipes are also baker's and brewer's yeast-free except for Leek and Red Pepper Salad, and Warm Beet Salad.

Quick, Crunchy Alfalfa Sprout Salad M

Yield: 2 servings

Alfalfa sprouts are particularly good served as a salad with a sunflower seed topping. This combination makes a delightfully light, crunchy summer salad.

2 tablespoons fresh lemon or lime juice	2 tablespoons hulled, toasted sunflower seeds
2 cups (4 ounces) alfalfa sprouts	

Pour the lemon or lime juice over sprouts and toss. Sprinkle seeds on top.

Squash Salad with Sesame Dressing M

Yield: 2 servings

The accent of ginger and sesame lends an Asian flavor to this unusual combination of vegetables. A satisfying dish that can be served as a meal in itself, this salad also is a wonderful complement to chicken, turkey, veal, or fish.

1 cup baked spaghetti
    squash*
1/2 cup julienned zucchini
1/2 cup julienned carrot
2 to 3 tablespoons
    julienned scallion
3/4 teaspoon fresh
    minced ginger (optional)

1 1/2 teaspoons fresh
    lemon or lime juice
1 teaspoon sesame oil
    (Japanese or other
    Asian)
1 teaspoon oil

1. Combine the squash, zucchini, carrot, scallion, and ginger in a bowl.
2. Place the lemon or lime juice in another bowl. Combine the oils. Slowly pour the oils into the juice, whisking constantly until the mixture is thick and cloudy.
3. Add the dressing to the squash mixture and toss. Serve within 2 hours so the vegetables remain crunchy. Chill if not served immediately.

*To bake a 3-pound spaghetti squash, split it in half horizontally and bake in a 400°F oven for 1 hour or until tender. Remove from the oven and cool. Remove the pulp with the tines of a fork. The remaining baked squash can be served as is or sautéed. Serve immediately or chill for a few days and reheat before serving.

Leek and Red Pepper Salad R, M

Yield: 2 servings

Rarely do so few ingredients offer such an attractive and mouth-watering package. These vegetables are sautéed quickly so that they retain their nutrients: potassium and vitamins A and C. This salad is particularly good served with roasted poultry or meat or cold poached fish.

1 teaspoon oil
1½ teaspoons thinly
  sliced garlic
2 cups (2 medium)
  ½-inch slices of leek

1 cup (2 medium)
  julienned sweet red
  pepper
2 teaspoons red wine
  vinegar

1. Heat nonstick sauté pan and add the oil. Add the garlic and sauté over low heat for 1 minute or until it smells pungent. (Remove the garlic with a slotted spoon if a milder flavor is desired.)
2. Add the leeks and separate the layers, for uniform cooking, while sautéing for 1 minute or until barely translucent. Add the red pepper and sauté for 1 minute.
3. Add the vinegar and sauté for 30 to 60 minutes or until the fumes are boiled off.
4. Transfer to a bowl to cool. Cover tightly and chill for 2 to 24 hours. Stir once to uniformly distribute vinaigrette.

Warm Beet Salad, R, M

Yield: 4 servings

This salad of warmed beets served with sautéed beet leaves uses its main ingredient with a minimum of waste. Although virtually ignored, beet leaves have a "meaty" texture and delicious flavor that make them most satisfying. This is a great dish because it is tasty, economical, and nutritious. When you serve this salad, you'll no longer have to command, "Eat your beets!" Your family will eat them with relish.

2 cups (1 pound) fresh beets, steamed*
3 tablespoons Mustard Vinaigrette Dressing (page 186)

3 cups beet greens, packed, stems removed
1 teaspoon dairy-free low-fat margarine

1. While still warm, peel and julienne the steamed beets. Toss with the vinaigrette. Reserve.
2. Bring water to a boil in a saucepan and immerse the fresh beet leaves in it. Blanch for 20 seconds. Drain and sauté immediately.
3. Heat a nonstick sauté pan, melt the margarine, and sauté the beet greens for 2 minutes or until they are just limp but still retain their vibrant color.
4. Arrange the sautéed beet leaves in a ring on individual serving plates. Mound the beets in the center of each ring and serve.

*Purchase young beets (1¾ pounds or 6 to 8 medium beets) with leaves attached. Select the best young, crisp leaves you can find; avoid leaves that are limp and starting to deteriorate.

Legume and Grain Salads

All of the recipes in the Legume and Grain Salad section are soy-free, cane sugar-free, egg-free, wheat-free, and baker's and brewer's yeast-free. All of the recipes are also corn-free and cow's milk-free except for the Tex-Mex Bean Salad unless its garnish is omitted.

Red Beans and Rice Salad M

Yield: 2 to 4 servings

This hearty combination of red kidney beans and rice is high in protein, phosphorus, and potassium and is low in fat. It is a satisfying meal in itself and is also an excellent accompaniment to warm or cold roast lamb or lean veal.

2 cups (1 19-ounce can) cooked red kidney beans

1 cup cooked long-grain brown rice (1/3 cup raw rice)

2 tablespoons chopped red onion

1/2 cup (3 ounces) diced pimiento

1/2 teaspoon minced garlic

3/4 teaspoon ground coriander

1/2 teaspoon ground cumin

Freshly ground black pepper to taste

1 1/2 teaspoons fresh lime or lemon juice

1 teaspoon oil

1. Mix the red beans, rice, vegetables, and seasonings in a bowl. Pour the lime or lemon juice into another bowl. Slowly pour in the oil, whisking constantly, until the mixture is thick and cloudy.
2. Add the dressing to the bean mixture and toss. Cover tightly and chill for at least 2 hours; stir once. This salad can be chilled for up to 2 days.

Vegetarian Delight M

Yield: 2 to 4 servings

This medley of warm black-eyed peas, rice, and spinach makes a great vegetarian dish, one that is delicious as well as nutritious.

2 cups (1 19-ounce can) cooked black-eyed peas

¾ cup cooked long-grain brown rice (¼ cup raw rice)

2 tablespoons chopped red onion

1 cup packed fresh spinach, chopped

½ cup (3 ounces) diced pimiento

½ teaspoon minced garlic

¾ teaspoon ground coriander

½ teaspoon ground cumin

1½ teaspoons fresh lime or lemon juice

Freshly ground black pepper to taste

1. In a nonstick pan heat the peas, rice, vegetables, garlic, and spices until warm.
2. Pour the lime or lemon juice onto the warm mixture and toss. Season to taste with the black pepper. Serve immediately.

Tabouleh Salad E, R, M

Yield: 4 servings

Although it is usually made with bulgur wheat, this tabouleh salad uses pearl barley for a delicious mix of moist, chewy grain and crisp vegetables. Tabouleh Salad is very nutritious, high in phosphorus, potassium, calcium, and vitamins A and C. It can easily be made in advance and is great for picnics.

1½ cups cooked pearl barley (½ cup dried pearl barley)
¼ cup diced sweet red pepper
¼ cup diced green pepper
¼ cup diced cucumber
3 tablespoons chopped scallion

3 tablespoons chopped parsley
¼ cup diced seeded plum tomatoes
4 tablespoons Tomato Juice Salad Dressing (page 182)
Freshly ground black pepper to taste

1. Place all ingredients in a bowl, toss and season to taste.
2. Chill for at least 1 hour. Stir once. Tabouleh Salad can be chilled for up to 2 days.

Vegetable-Rice Salad R, M

Yield: 4 servings

This chilled rice salad studded with fresh vegetables is a great way to use extra raw vegetables or leftover cooked rice. Light and refreshing, Vegetable-Rice Salad is particularly good served with chilled poached fish. It also makes an excellent vegetarian lunch that is easy to take to work or school.

*1½ cups cooked long-
grain brown rice (½
cup raw rice)*
*⅓ cup chopped seeded
tomato*
⅓ cup diced radish

⅓ cup diced cucumber
*2 tablespoons chopped
scallion*
*2 tablespoons Tomato
Juice Salad Dressing
(page 182)*

Garnish (optional)

*Chopped fresh parsley or
whole coriander leaves*

1. Combine rice and vegetables in a bowl; add dressing and toss.
2. Cover tightly and refrigerate at least 2 hours (or up to 24 hours) so the flavors blend. Stir once during this time. If desired, sprinkle the parsley or coriander on top before serving.

VARIATIONS: 1. This is an extremely versatile salad and you can make substitutions to suit your taste. Chopped black olives, zucchini, green pepper, and asparagus are a good variation. Just remember that the ratio is 1 cup fresh vegetables to 1½ cups cooked rice.

2. Herbs can be used to change the flavor of this salad. Use 1 teaspoon fresh thyme, basil, or oregano or ¼ teaspoon dried.

3. Pearl barley may be substituted for the rice. Use 1½ cups cooked barley (½ cup raw).

Tex-Mex Bean Salad, R, M

Yield: 2 servings

This pinto bean salad exemplifies one of America's great regional cuisines—Tex-Mex. Serve it with grilled or barbecued chicken, and try it as a welcome change from ordinary refried beans.

*2 cups (1 19-ounce can)
cooked pinto beans or
kidney beans*
*½ cup diced green
pepper*
*½ cup chopped seeded
plum tomatoes*
*4 teaspoons minced
scallion, leek, or
shallot*
*2 teaspoons thinly sliced
fresh chili pepper
(optional)*

*½ teaspoon minced
garlic*
*¼ teaspoon ground
coriander*
*⅛ teaspoon ground
cumin*
*¼ teaspoon minced lime
zest*
*1½ teaspoons fresh lime
juice*

Garnish (optional)

*½ cup (4 ounces) shredded
low-fat Cheddar or low-
fat mozzarella cheese*

Tostaditas

1. Combine all ingredients except the lime juice and toss. Serve immediately or cover tightly and chill for a few hours. Stir once to distribute spices uniformly.
2. If using the garnish, sprinkle the cheese on top of the salad just before serving. Warm the tostadita chips in a 300°F oven for 10 minutes and serve in a decorative bowl or basket.

White Bean Salad, E, R, M

Yield: 2 servings

White beans are one of the most popular legumes. Usually served as one of many ingredients in soups, stews, and cassoulets, here these beans are given star billing as a salad to emphasize how delicious and versatile they really are. This salad is economical to make and very nutritious with its balance of protein and carbohydrate. It can easily be prepared in advance, and is great for a picnic.

2 cups (1 19-ounce can) cooked white kidney beans (cannellini beans) or Great Northern beans

⅓ cup diced sweet red pepper

⅓ cup diced green pepper

1 tablespoon finely chopped onion or scallion

⅜ teaspoon minced garlic

2 tablespoon Citrus Salad Dressing (page 183)

Freshly ground black pepper to taste

1. Combine all ingredients in a bowl and toss.
2. Season to taste. Cover tightly and refrigerate. This salad is best if left to marinate for a few hours so the flavors blend. It can be kept chilled for up to 2 days.

Vegetable Dishes

All of the recipes in the Vegetable section are corn-free, soy-free, cane sugar-free, egg-free, cow's milk-free, and wheat-free. All of the recipes are baker's and brewer's yeast-free except for Stir-Fried Summer Vegetables with Coriander and Basil.

Braised Escarole M

Yield: 2 servings

This quickly prepared and delicious side dish is excellent with chicken and fish.

2 teaspoons oil
¼ cup thinly sliced
  scallions
2 teaspoons thinly sliced
  garlic

4 cups (8 ounces)
  2-inch slices of
  escarole

Heat a nonstick pan until warm and add the oil. Sauté the scallions and garlic for 15 seconds. Add the escarole and sauté for approximately 1 to 2 minutes or until it becomes barely limp. Cover and simmer over low heat for 3 to 5 minutes or until barely soft. If the escarole becomes too dry, add 2 to 4 tablespoons water or broth or it may burn.

Stir-Fried Summer Vegetables with Coriander and Basil M

Yield: 4 servings

Brilliant color and crisp texture characterize this mélange of ripe summer vegetables. Stir-frying retains the color, texture, and nutrients, and the flavors are accented with coriander and fresh basil. This is an excellent accompaniment to simply prepared chicken and fish dishes.

2 teaspoons oil
1 cup (1 narrow medium) roll-cut zucchini*
1 cup (1 narrow medium) roll-cut yellow squash*
1¼ cups (1 medium) 1-inch cubed sweet red pepper
1 cup (1 medium) 1-inch cubed Spanish onion

⅛ cup thinly sliced garlic (for mild flavor) or minced garlic (for strong flavor)
1 teaspoon kalounji (black onion seed; optional)
2 teaspoons dried ground coriander
⅓ cup shredded fresh basil, packed, or ¾ teaspoon dried
⅛ cup red wine vinegar

1. Heat a nonstick pan or wok and add the oil. Add the zucchini and stir-fry for 2 minutes. Add the yellow squash and stir-fry for 1 minute. Add the red pepper

*To roll-cut the two squashes, slice diagonally every ¾ inch *but* roll the squash a quarter of its circumference before each slice as follows: slice, roll one-quarter, slice, roll one-quarter, etc. The pieces will be rather triangular in shape with much of the interior exposed to facilitate quick cooking. This is an excellent Chinese technique used for firm vegetables; they cook quickly to uniform tenderness while retaining essential nutrients.

and stir-fry for 45 seconds. Add the onion and stir-fry for 15 seconds, separating the layers to facilitate even cooking of the onion.

2. Add the garlic and stir-fry until pungent, about 15 seconds. Add the kalounji, if using, and the coriander and stir-fry until the vegetables are just tender, 2 to 3 minutes.

3. Add the basil. Add the vinegar and stir-fry until the vinegar fumes have evaporated, approximately 10 seconds. Total stir-frying time should be about 8 minutes. Remove from the heat. Serve warm or at room temperature.

Carrot Puree on a Bed of Leeks M

Yield: 2 servings

This carrot and leek dish is so pretty and delicious that it belongs on fine restaurant menus, yet, it can easily be made in a matter of minutes at home. A wonderful dinner party dish that goes particularly well with beef, veal, or fish, it is also a satisfying meal by itself. As an added benefit, it is high in vitamin A and potassium.

*1⅓ cups trimmed and
    unpeeled carrots, cut
    in 2-inch sections
1⅓ cups sliced leek*
2 teaspoons dairy-free,*

*low-fat margarine,
    divided
Freshly ground white
    pepper and nutmeg to
    taste*

Garnish (optional)

*2 tablespoons freshly snipped
    dill or parsley*

1. Steam the carrots until their centers are just tender when pierced with a fork. (The steaming time will be approximately 10 minutes for young carrots and 18 minutes for mature carrots.) Transfer to a blender or food processor, and chop until finely minced or smoothly pureed. Season to taste. Keep warm.
2. Heat a nonstick pan and melt the margarine. Sauté the leeks 4 to 5 minutes over medium heat until barely tender and limp, retaining bright color. Season to taste.

---

* Use only the stalk of the leek and save the leaves for another dish or for broth. Trim off the roots, split the leek lengthwise, and rinse under cold running water to remove residue grit. Drain and pat dry. Slice horizontally into ½-inch slices.

3. On individual serving plates, arrange a ring of leeks and place a large dollop of carrot puree in the center of the ring. Garnish with a light sprinkling of fresh dill or parsley if desired.

VARIATION: Substitute steamed pureeed white turnips (1⅓ cups), which are high in potassium, for the carrots.

Steamed Carrots with Dill M

Yield: 2 servings

These carrots, cooked until just tender and accented with dill, are light and refreshing and are especially good with chicken or fish. Carrots, a fantastic source of vitamin A, are also high in potassium, and steaming retains nutrients as well as delicious flavor.

2 cups (6 medium) carrots   *1 tablespoon fresh dill*
Freshly ground white   *or 1¼ teaspoons dried*
* pepper to taste*

1. Steam carrots until tender. The steaming time will be approximately 10 minutes for young carrots and 18 minutes for mature carrots.
2. Transfer the carrots to a serving plate and sprinkle with dill. Season to taste.

Sautéed Okra E, R, M

Yield: 2 servings

These little green pods seem to evoke strong feelings, perhaps because of their unusual texture as a result of pickling or stewing. However, sautéing them produces a different effect. My husband, a Southerner, showed me this "down-home" method that makes okra a delicate treat that is tender inside and lightly crisped outside. Quite low in calories, okra is high in vitamin A, potassium, and calcium. Sautéed okra is a delicious complement to casseroles and stews as well as simple beef, poultry, and fish dishes.

*2 cups (10 ounces)
    trimmed, ½-inch
    slices of okra*
⅛ cup flour (oat, rye)
*Freshly ground white
    pepper to taste*

*2 teaspoons dairy-free
    low-fat margarine*

1. Roll the sliced okra in flour and pepper to taste until well coated.
2. Heat a nonstick pan until warm. Melt the margarine. Over medium-high heat, sauté the okra for 8 to 10 minutes or until tender with crisp, light-brown edges.

Stir-Fried Snow Peas
with Water Chestnuts E, R, M

Yield: 2 servings

These two vegetables have crispness and natural sweetness that complement not only all of the Chinese cuisines, but many other cuisines as well. They make an outstanding accompaniment to fish and chicken and are excellent with roast beef or steak.

2 cups (30) snow peas
1½ teaspoon oil
¼ cup (4) thinly sliced
  water chestnuts, fresh
  or canned

Freshly ground white
  pepper to taste

1. Rinse the snow peas and trim both ends. If the snow peas are to be left whole, remove the strings along the straight edge. Otherwise, cut in half.
2. Heat a nonstick pan or wok until hot and add the oil. Add the snow peas and stir-fry for 20 seconds. Add the water chestnuts and stir-fry for 30 seconds or until both vegetables are barely tender while retaining a little crispness. Add the white pepper to taste. Serve.

Steamed Asparagus with Tarragon E, R, M

Yield: 2 servings

The harbinger of spring, asparagus is best when simply prepared. Accenting it with tarragon produces a flavor that is particularly complementary to fish and chicken dishes. Asparagus is a good source of vitamin E.

8 ounces (10 thick to 16 thin spears) fresh asparagus spears

4 teaspoons fresh tarragon or 1½ teaspoons dried

Freshly ground white pepper to taste

1. Wash and trim the asparagus. Peel the stalk if desired.
2. Steam the asparagus until barely tender (about 4 to 6 minutes for thin stalks, 8 to 10 minutes for thick).
3. To serve, sprinkle the tarragon over the steamed asparagus.

Broiled Tomato with Herbs E, R, M

Yield: 2 servings

Broiling brings out the luscious flavor of ripe tomatoes, and the herb accent creates a special side dish, especially with broiled fish, poultry, and meats. In addition, tomatoes are very high in vitamin A and contain a substantial amount of potassium and amino acids.

*1 large ripe beefsteak
  tomato*
*2 teaspoons fresh
  rosemary, oregano,
  and/or basil or ½
  teaspoon dried*

*Freshly ground black
  pepper to taste*

1. Split the tomato in half, horizontally. Do not peel or remove the core. Rub the herbs on the cut surface of both halves. Add the pepper, if using, and mix. Place the broiler pan 4 inches from the heat source. Preheat the broiler.
2. Line a metal pie plate or cake pan with aluminum foil. Place the tomato halves on the plate or pan with the cut surface up.
3. Broil for 5 to 8 minutes or until very hot.

Broiled Sweet Red Pepper E, R, M

Yield: 2 servings

Light broiling releases the fragrant flavor of these red peppers. Serve this simple savory dish with broiled fish, meats, or poultry.

2 large sweet red peppers

1. Place the broiler pan 4 inches away from the heat source. Preheat the broiler. Remove the stems, seeds, and pith and split lengthwise into quarters.
2. Place skin side up on the broiler pan and cook for 2 minutes. Turn over and cook for another 2 minutes. (Do not overcook or the red peppers will be too soft. They should retain a slight crunchy texture).

Broiled Onion E, R, M

Yield: 2 servings

This is a simple yet delicious vegetable side dish. Onions are high in phosphorus, potassium, magnesium, calcium, and amino acids, and low in calories.

1 large Bermuda or red onion, peeled

1. Cut the onion in half vertically. Cut the onion halves into ¾-inch-thick slices. Separate the slices. Place the broiler pan 4 inches from the heat source. Preheat the broiler.
2. Arrange the slices in a single layer and broil for 5 to 7 minutes, or until browned at the edges but still slightly crisp. Turn the slices over once during the broiling. Serve immediately.

Broiled Eggplant E, R, M

Yield: 2 servings

For a special treat, try broiling eggplant instead of sautéeing or frying it. Simple to prepare, broiled eggplant can either be served as is or pureed into a cream that is rich in taste but not in calories.

*1 medium eggplant,
trimmed and quar-
tered lengthwise
Fresh or dried oregano
to taste*

*Ground cumin and
white pepper to taste
Fresh lemon juice to
taste*

1. Place the broiler pan 4 inches from the heat source. Preheat the broiler.
2. Broil the eggplant quarters for 10 to 15 minutes, turning once to brown evenly. The eggplant is done when it is soft and exuding some water on its surface. Serve as is, unpeeled, or peel, drain between sheets of absorbent paper, and puree for a smooth, creamy eggplant side dish. Before serving, season to taste.

Sautéed Cabbage with Onions E, R, M

Yield: 2 servings

Cabbage is often unappreciated and under-utilized because so many people cook it for hours or serve it pickled as sauerkraut or stuffed and wrapped into rolls. Yet cabbage is delicious cooked quickly so that it retains a little crunch and a lot of character. If you have not made sautéed cabbage before, try this recipe. It is amazingly low in calories and high in vitamin A, potassium, and calcium.

*1 tablespoon dairy-free,
    low-fat margarine*
*2½ cups ½-inch slices
    of cabbage, packed*
*½ cup ¼-inch slices of
    onion*

*Freshly ground white or
    black pepper to taste*

1. Heat a nonstick pan until warm and melt the margarine.
2. Add the cabbage and sauté for 5 minutes over medium heat or until it is just limp. Add the onion and sauté for 3 minutes or until it is translucent and limp. Season to taste.

Grain Dishes

All of the receeipes in the Grain Dishes section are corn-free, cow's milk-free, and cane sugar-free. All of the recipes are egg-free except for the Rye Spätzle. All are soy-free, wheat-free, and baker's and brewer's yeast-free except for Eight Varieties Fried Rice.

Boiled Millet E, R, M

Yield: 1 cup

Millet, native to Asia and a principal grain of Europe, tastes like a cross between wheat and corn. It is great warm as a breakfast cereal or as a side dish for stews and casseroles, and is high in protein, niacin, phosphorus, potassium, calcium, iron, and magnesium.

⅓ cup raw whole millet   *additional ⅛ cup*
1 cup water with an   *reserved*

Place the millet and 1 cup water into a small saucepan. Bring the water to a boil, reduce to a simmer, and cook for 2 to 3 minutes. Cover and continue to simmer for 25 to 30 minutes, or until tender. Stir occasionally to prevent sticking. (Add up to ⅛ cup water if needed during the simmering.)

Boiled Pearl Barley E, R, M

Yield: 1 cup

Boiled pearl barley is a wonderful alternative to rice, wheat pasta, and hot cereals. You can also use it as a side dish with roasted meats as well as in salads and soups. Barley is high in protein, phosphorus, potassium, calcium, and magnesium.

⅓ cup raw pearl barley   *additional ½ cup*
1¼ cups water with an   *reserved*

Put the barley and 1¼ cups water into a small saucepan. Bring the water to a boil, reduce to a simmer, and cook for 2 to 3 minutes. Cover and continue to simmer for 25 to 30 minutes, or until tender. Stir occasionally to prevent sticking. (Add up to ½ cup water if needed during the simmering.)

Boiled Buckwheat Groats or Kasha E, R, M

Yield: 1 cup

Buckwheat groats or kasha is used extensively throughout Asia and Central Europe; it can be served as a warm cereal or as a side dish. Buckwheat is high in potassium, magnesium, and amino acids, and low in fat.

*½ cup raw buckwheat
  groats or kasha
1¼ cups water or broth
  (chicken, turkey,*
*beef, veal, vegetable)
  with an additional ¼
  cup reserved*

Put the groats or kasha and 1¼ cups water into a small saucepan. Bring the water to a boil, reduce to a simmer and cook for 3 to 5 minutes or until tender. Stir occasionally to prevent sticking. (Add up to ¼ cup water if needed during the simmering.)

Boiled Long-Grain Brown Rice E, R, M

Yield: 1 cup

Brown rice is simply white rice that still has its outer husk. More nutritious than white rice, brown rice is high in protein, phosphorus, potassium, calcium, magnesium, selenium, and amino acids.

⅓ cup raw long-grain brown   additional ⅛ cup
  rice   reserved
1¼ cups water with an

Put the rice and 1¼ cups water into a small saucepan. Bring the water to a boil, reduce to a simmer, and cook for 2 to 3 minutes. Cover and continue to simmer for 25 to 30 minutes, or until tender. Stir occasionally to prevent sticking. (Add up to ⅛ cup water if needed during the simmering.)

Eight Varieties Fried Rice M

Yield: 2 servings

This version of the versatile Cantonese dish uses leftover rice, which has a firm texture. The recipe can easily be adjusted to individual preference, and leftover ingredients as well as fresh ones can be used. Eight Varieties Fried Rice provides a variety of tastes and textures and is very nutritious, offering a balance of protein, fat, and carbohydrate.

2 cups leftover cooked long-grain brown rice

3 dried Chinese black mushrooms, soaked in hot water and squeezed of excess water, chopped, or 3 fresh sliced mushrooms

3 water chestnuts, fresh or canned, chopped

¼ cup raw peas

2 scallions, thickly sliced

½ cup bean sprouts

1½ tablespoons oil

½ cup thinly sliced bok choy or celery

½ cup chopped, skinned, boneless chicken

6 (6 ounces) raw shrimp, shelled, cleaned, and chopped

5 teaspoons light soy sauce or chicken broth

1 tablespoon oyster sauce (optional)

Freshly ground white pepper to taste

1. Boil the rice 1 day in advance. Refrigerate. Bring to room temperature before stir-frying.
2. Combine the mushrooms, water chestnuts, and peas. Combine the scallions and bean sprouts.
3. Heat a nonstick, wok until hot and add the oil. Add the

mushrooms, water chestnuts, and peas, and stir-fry for 20 seconds. Add the bok choy or celery and stir-fry for 10 seconds. Add the chicken and stir-fry until it loses its pink color, about 10 seconds. Add the shrimp and stir-fry until they turn pink, about 10 seconds. Add the rice and stir-fry for 20 seconds. Add the scallions and bean sprouts and mix. Add the soy sauce or chicken broth (and oyster sauce) and stir-fry for 20 seconds. Season to taste with the white pepper.

VARIATION: Any leftover meat may be used, as well as any vegetables. The cooking technique remains the same. The ratio is 2 cups cooked rice, 1 cup meat, poultry, or shellfish, and 1¾ cups vegetables.

Rye Spätzle R, M

Yield: 2 servings

Spätzle are marvelous little dumpling-noodles typical of
Central European cuisine. They are terrific with stews or
any other braised dishes that have gravy. For those of you
with wheat allergies, this rye version is just as good as the
classic wheat spätzle.

1 cup (4.25 ounces) rye   *⅓ to ½ cup boiling water*
  flour   *¼ teaspoon baking soda*
3 large egg yolks,
  lightly beaten

1. Place flour in a bowl and pour in the beaten egg
   yolks while mixing with a fork. Pour in the ⅓ cup
   water and continue mixing until a smooth dough is
   formed. (It should be the consistency of cookie
   dough. Add additional water, 1 teaspoon at a time,
   if necessary.) Add the baking soda and mix well.
   Cover and let rest at room temperature for 30 to 60
   minutes.
2. Bring water to a boil in a large pot. Using a fork, scoop
   up a small amount of dough and hold it over the boiling
   water. Cut small pieces off with a sharp knife and let
   fall into the water. (Or use a cookie press with the
   spätzle plate.) Boil for 1 to 2 minutes or until tender.
   Drain.

Dressings and Sauces

All of the recipes in the Dressings and Sauces section are egg-free, corn-free, cane sugar-free, wheat-free, and cow's milk-free. All of the recipes are also soy-free, except for the Soybean Mayonnaise and Fluffy Soybean Mayonnaise. All are baker's and brewer's yeast-free except for Warm Garlic Dressing if vinegar is used.

Tomato Juice Salad Dressing E, R, M

Yield: 2 servings

This light yet flavorful salad dressing is deliciously satisfying whether you're on a diet or not.

2 tablespoons tomato juice
1 tablespoon water
1 thin slice garlic
  (optional)
Ground cayenne pepper
  to taste (optional)
Up to 1 tablespoon fresh

or ½ teaspoon dried
of the following singly
or in combination:
basil, chives, coriander
leaves, dill, marjo-
ram, oregano, parsley,
thyme

Mix the juice and water together in a bowl. Add the garlic, if using, herbs, and/or spices desired and mix. If possible, chill, covered, in the refrigerator for 30 to 60 minutes before serving so there is time for the herbs and/or spices to flavor the salad dressing. (If using the garlic slice, remove before tossing the salad.)

Citrus Salad Dressing E, R, M

Yield: 2 servings

Although similar to plain vinegar, Citrus Salad Dressing is an infinitely more appealing and tasty way to perk up a salad.

1½ tablespoons fresh lemon, lime, or grapefruit juice
3½ to 4 teaspoons water
1 slice fresh garlic (optional)
Up to 1 tablespoon fresh or ½ teaspoon dried

of the following singly or in combination: basil, chives, coriander leaves, marjoram, mint, oregano, parsley, thyme
Ground cumin to taste (optional)

Mix the juice and water together in a bowl. Add the garlic, if using, herbs, and/or spices desired and mix. If possible, chill, covered, in the refrigerator for 30 to 60 minutes before serving so there is time for the herbs and/or spices to flavor the salad dressing. (If using the garlic slice, remove before tossing the salad.)

VARIATION: Substitute fresh orange juice and reduce the water to 2½ to 3 teaspoons.

Ancho Sauce M

Yield: 8 servings

This luscious sauce is made from sun-dried ancho chili peppers, herbs, and tomatoes. Its subtle richness complements chicken dishes and is excellent with broiled chicken or Chicken Satés (see page 194).

*2 ounces (4 to 5) dried
    ancho peppers*
*¼ cup (1.5 ounces)
    ground blanched
    almonds or brazil nuts,
    toasted*
*1 small garlic clove
    (optional)*
*⅛ teaspoon ground
    cinnamon*
*⅛ teaspoon ground
    cloves*

*¾ teaspoon fresh
    oregano or ¼ tea-
    spoon dried*
*¾ cup chicken broth or
    water, divided*
*⅓ cup fresh orange,
    tangerine, or tangelo
    juice*
*2½ tablespoons tomato
    concentrate or paste*

1. Roast peppers in a 350° F oven for 2 minutes or until soft and leathery. *Do not* overroast or the peppers will become bitter; if they become brittle, taste for any bitterness. Split and remove pith, seeds, and stem.
2. Tear the peppers into small pieces and chop in a blender or food processor (use the steel chopping blade). Add the almonds or brazil nuts, garlic, if used, spices, and herb, and chop until pureed. Pour in ⅔ cup of the broth or water and juice and blend for 5 minutes or until thick, smooth, and rust-colored. Add the tomato concentrate and mix well.

3. Heat the sauce in a nonstick pot and cook over low heat, stirring constantly, for 5 minutes or until thick. Add the remaining broth or water to thin if necessary. Serve or refrigerate for up to 2 days or freeze up to 1 month and thaw overnight in the refrigerator. Simply reheat before serving.

Mustard Vinaigrette Dressing R, M

Yield: 4 servings

This dressing is completely oil-free and is delicious on
leafy green salads.

2 teaspoons Dijon mustard
6 tablespoons broth
  (chicken, turkey, or
  vegetable)
½ teaspoon minced
  fresh chervil, parsley,
  or basil or ⅛ teaspoon
  dried

1 tablespoon red or
  white wine vinegar
1 teaspoon fresh lemon
  juice (optional)
¼ teaspoon freshly
  ground pepper

Mix all the ingredients together in a bowl. Chill, covered,
in the refrigerator for 1 hour before serving, so there is
time for the flavors to blend.

Warm Garlic Dressing M

Yield: 2 servings

Warm garlic dressing is especially good poured over steamed broccoli, cauliflower, artichokes, asparagus, and green beans. Heating the garlic extracts its flavor so that it blends with the oil to make an aromatic dressing. This is a quick way to change ordinary steamed vegetables into a most flavorful dish.

1 teaspoon thinly sliced
  garlic
1 teaspoon oil
1½ tablespoons red or
white wine vinegar,
lime juice, or lemon
juice

1. Place ingredients in a small saucepan, cover (dressing may splatter when heated), and warm over low heat for 5 minutes. The garlic will be pungent when done, and the vinegar, if used, will have lost its sharpness.
2. Remove garlic slices if desired. Pour immediately over freshly steamed vegetables.

VARIATIONS: 1. Substitute sliced onion or scallion for the garlic in the same amount.

2. Rosemary, oregano, or marjoram may be added for flavor. Use up to 1 teaspoon fresh or ¼ teaspoon dried, singly or blended.

Soybean Mayonnaise R, M

Yield: 4 to 6 servings

Soybean mayonnaise is a luscious substitute for regular
egg mayonnaise. It is smooth and creamy and can be used
as a sauce, dip, or salad dressing.

6 ounces fresh hard   *3 tablespoons oil*
  soybean curd (tofu)
5 teaspoons fresh lemon
  or lime juice

1. Cut the soybean curd into ½-inch-thick slices,
   place between layers of a cotton kitchen towel and
   gently pat so most of the water is absorbed.
2. Transfer curd to a dry towel and wrap and twist to
   wring out excess water. Gently knead the curd during
   this process. (It is all right if the curd breaks apart
   because it will be pureed later.)
3. Put the soybean curd in a blender or food processor
   (use the steel chopping blade) and puree. Pour in the
   lemon or lime juice and blend for 30 seconds. Slowly
   pour in the oil, 1 tablespoon at a time, and continue to
   blend for 2 to 3 minutes or until creamy and emulsified.
4. Store in a tightly sealed jar and chill up to 4 days. As
   the mayonnaise ages, the acidity of the lemon or lime
   juice will become more assertive, but pleasantly so.

Fluffy Soybean Mayonnaise R, M

Yield: 4 servings

This version is similar to soybean mayonnaise in flavor. However, since silken soybean curd is used, the result is fluffier—more like a dense whipped cream.

6 ounces fresh silken soybean curd (tofu)

2 teaspoons fresh lemon or lime juice
2 tablespoons oil

1. Cut the soybean curd into ½-inch-thick slices, place between layers of a cotton kitchen towel and gently pat so most of the water is absorbed.
2. Transfer curd to a dry towel and wrap and twist to wring out excess water. Gently knead the curd during this process. (It is all right if the curd breaks apart because it will be pureed later.)
3. Put the soybean curd in a blender or food processor (use the steel chopping blade) and puree. Pour in the lemon or lime juice and blend for 30 seconds. Slowly pour in the oil, 1 tablespoon at a time, and continue to blend for 2 to 3 minutes or until creamy, emulsified, and fluffy.
4. If a light and fluffy mayonnaise is desired, use within 1 hour of making. If a denser mayonnaise is preferred, store in a tightly sealed jar and chill up to 4 days. Drain off any residual water that may collect on the top before serving.

Main Dishes

All of the recipes in the Main Dishes section are cane sugar-free. All are corn-free except for Römertopf Roast Chicken with Herbs and Chicken with Bourbon Sauce, unless the cornstarch is omitted. All are soy-free except for Turkey Salad with Raisins and wheat-free except for Chinese Lettuce Packages, Stir-Fried Beef with Broccoli and Mushrooms, and Chinese Steamed Red Snapper. Turkey Hash is also wheat-free if a different flour is substituted for wheat flour. All the recipes are egg-free except for Tuna Niçoise unless the egg is omitted. All are cow's milk-free except for Linguine with 30-Minute Fresh Tomato Sauce and Spaghetti with Bolognese Sauce unless the cow's milk cheese topping is omitted. All are baker's and brewer's yeast-free except for Chicken with Bourbon Sauce, Chinese Lettuce Packages, Stir-Fried Beef with Broccoli and Mushrooms, and Chinese Steamed Red Snapper.

Millet-Baked Chicken M

Yield: 4 servings

Replacing the usual breadcrumb, egg, and milk coating with millet meal makes this baked chicken crispier. In addition, millet-baked chicken is easier to make and lower in calories than the usual version.

2½-pound young broiler,   *Fresh or dried thyme,*
  chopped into 16   *oregano, basil, or*
  pieces   *sage to taste*
½ cup millet meal
Freshly ground black
  pepper to taste

1. Remove the chicken from the refrigerator 30 minutes before baking and peel off the skin to substantially reduce calories, fat, and cholesterol.
2. Mix the millet meal, pepper, and herbs together in a bowl. Rinse the chicken under warm running water, drain, and roll in the millet meal mixture until well coated. Preheat the oven to 450° F.
3. Put a cooling rack on a baking sheet so that any rendered fat can drip into the pan during baking. Arrange the chicken pieces on top of the rack. Place the chicken in the center of the oven, reduce the heat to 425° F, and bake for 15 to 20 minutes. Remove from the oven, turn each piece over, and continue baking for another 15 to 20 minutes. Remove and drain on absorbent paper and serve immediately.

Römertopf® Roast Chicken with Herbs E, R, M

Yield: 4 servings

This method of roasting produces one of the most delectable chickens. In just a little more than an hour's cooking time, the meat will be almost falling off the bone it's so tender and moist. In addition, chicken broth will be extracted from the bird during the roasting without ever adding any water or broth, yielding a pure essence of chicken that can be used to make a sauce or spooned over boiled pearl barley or rice as a delicious accompaniment.

2½-pound young broiler
2 tablespoons fresh
  tarragon, summer
  savory, or marjoram,
  used singly or blended,

or 1½ teaspoons dried
  (optional)
¼ teaspoon cornstarch
  (optional)

Always put the Römertopf in a COLD oven; do not preheat.

1. Soak the Römertopf pot and lid in warm water for 10 minutes. Drain.
2. Place the herb or herbs (if desired) in the cavity of the chicken and over the cavity's surface. Place the chicken in the pot, breast-down, and arrange giblets around it.
3. Put the pot and cover* in a cold oven and turn the heat to 500° F, leaving the pot uncovered for this stage. It should take 5 to 10 minutes for the oven to reach 500°F.

* The cover must go into the oven at this time so that it can heat along with the pot and the oven; simply put it on another rack. If it were put cold into a 500° F oven, the top would probably crack.

4. Begin timing the roasting of the chicken now by searing it at 500°F for 10 minutes. Turn the chicken over so that the breast is up and continue to sear for 10 minutes.

5. Cover the chicken and reduce the heat to 350°F. Roast for 40 to 50 minutes. The chicken should be very tender, almost falling off the bone.

6. Remove the giblets and reserve or discard. Drain the cavity of its juices into the pot. Transfer the chicken to a carving board and let rest for at least 10 to 15 minutes so the juice can be redistributed. Strain the juice from the pot and discard the rendered fat, if desired. Approximately ½ cup of juice should remain. (If more juice is desired, either add some HOT water during the last 20 minutes of roasting or add water or broth to the juice before warming.)

7. Scrape some of the herbs from the cavity of the bird into the juice. Warm the juice (thicken with ¼ teaspoon cornstarch mixed with 1 tablespoon water, if desired) and serve.

VARIATIONS: 1. Substitute ⅛ teaspoon arrowroot, potato starch, or water chestnut powder for the cornstarch.

2. For an individual serving, roast a chicken breast (5 to 6 ounces) with the Römertopf covered. Place in a cold oven and turn the heat to 350° F. It should take 3 to 5 minutes for the oven to reach 350° F. Then roast for 5 to 10 minutes. (If desired, add ½ cup broth halfway through cooking.)

Chicken Satés E, R, M

Yield: 2 servings

Satés are like small shish kebabs, the difference being that *satés* contain only meat. They have always been a hit with my cooking-school students because they are so easy to prepare and so good to eat—especially served with Ancho Sauce (a zippy Mexican chili sauce; see page 184). Make more than you think you'll need—they have a way of disappearing quickly.

**12-16 ounces skinned,
  boned chicken breasts,
  cut into 1-inch pieces**

Marinade

*¾ teaspoon fresh ground
  allspice*

*½ teaspoon fresh
  ground black pepper*

*1½ teaspoon fresh
  oregano or ½ tea-
  spoon dried*

*¾ teaspoon ground
  cumin*

*¾ teaspoon ground
  coriander*

*5 small garlic cloves,
  pressed (optional)*

1 teaspoon oil

*3 tablespoons fresh
  orange, tangerine, or
  tangelo juice*

**8 bamboo saté sticks or
  metal skewers**

1. Place the chicken in a bowl. Mix and add the marinade. Combine thoroughly. Cover tightly and chill for 4 to 24 hours so the meat will absorb some of the marinade's flavor. Stir once to distribute the flavor uniformly.

2. Soak the bamboo sticks in cold water for 1 hour so they do not burn during cooking.

3. Adjust the rack so the *satés* will be 4 inches from the heat source. Preheat the broiler or grill. Skewer the chicken loosely so all surfaces will get cooked.

4. Broil or grill the *satés* for 3 minutes, turn over, and grill for 2 minutes more. Serve immediately.

Chicken Cacciatore M

Yield: 2 to 4 servings

The chicken in this luscious, classic Northern Italian dish simmers gently until tender in a tomato sauce redolent with herbs. It should be served with rice, noodles, or pearl barley to absorb the sauce, which is far too good to waste. A perfect dinner party dish, Chicken Cacciatore can be made in advance.

2 teaspoons oil
½ cup chopped onion
2 teaspoons sliced garlic
¼ cup chopped fresh parsley
2 pounds skinned chicken, chopped into 16 pieces
2 cups chicken broth
2 cups (1 pound) chopped plum tomatoes

½ small dried bay leaf
3 tablespoons fresh basil or 1 teaspoon dried
1 carrot, cut into 2-inch sections
1 stalk celery, cut into 2-inch sections
Freshly ground allspice or black pepper to taste

1. Heat a nonstick casserole until warm and add the oil. Sauté the onoin for 1 minute over medium heat.
2. Add the garlic and parsley and sauté for 30 seconds.
3. Add the chicken and sear on all sides over medium heat for 5 minutes.
4. Add the broth, tomatoes, and herbs and mix well. Add the carrot and celery.
5. Bring to a boil for 1 minute, reduce to simmer, and cook for 2 hours, turning occasionally.

6. Skim the rendered chicken fat off the top of the sauce, if desired. Season to taste with allspice or pepper.
7. Serve immediately with boiled rice, boiled egg noodles, or boiled pearl barley (see page 175). Chicken Cacciatore can be refrigerated for up to 2 days. Warm over low heat for 15 minutes before serving.

Chinese Lettuce Packages M

Yield: 2 to 4 servings

These crispy packages, filled with a luscious mixture of meat and vegetables, make a well-balanced meal that is always a favorite in my cooking school. Chinese Lettuce Packages can be served as an appetizer or main dish and are a good dish for a party since guests can assemble their own.

1 head iceberg, romaine, or Bibb lettuce
12 ounces ground lean fresh skinned boneless chicken breasts
¼ teaspoon minced garlic
2 teaspoons shao-hsing wine or dry sherry
4 teaspoons light soy sauce, divided
⅔ cup diced celery
¾ cup (12) diced fresh or canned water chestnuts
⅓ cup diced bamboo shoots

½ cup (8 medium) dried black mushrooms, soaked in hot water and squeezed of excess water, stems removed, diced
2 teaspoons oil
1 to 2 tablespoons black beans, rinsed and slightly crushed (optional)
1 tablespoon oyster sauce (optional)

1. Separate, rinse, and dry the lettuce leaves. Arrange on a platter and chill until serving time.
2. Combine the chicken, garlic, wine or sherry, and 2 teaspoons soy sauce. Mix until well blended and re-

serve. Combine the celery, water chestnuts, bamboo shoots, and mushrooms, if using, and reserve.

3. Heat a nonstick wok or sauté pan until hot and add the oil. Stir-fry the mixture until the chicken loses its pink color, about 1 minute. Add the vegetable mixture and stir-fry for 1 minute. (If using the black beans, stir-fry with the vegetables.) Add 2 teaspoons soy sauce and stir-fry for 15 seconds. (If using the oyster sauce, add and blend). Transfer to a decorative bowl and serve with the chilled lettuce leaves.

4. To assemble the Chinese Lettuce Packages, simply put some of the meat mixture in a lettuce leaf and roll up or fold.

Chicken with Bourbon Sauce M

Yield: 2 servings

These tender breasts of chicken laced with a lusicous bourbon sauce make an elegant meal in a matter of minutes.

2 teaspoons dairy-free, low-fat margarine, divided
2 chicken breasts (6 to 8 ounces each), boned and skinned
¼ cup chopped onion
⅔ cup (3 ounces) sliced fresh mushrooms

½ cup chicken broth
¼ cup bourbon
1 teaspoon cornstarch mixed with 2 teaspoons chicken broth (optional)

1. Heat a nonstick sauté pan and melt 1 teaspoon margarine. Over medium heat sear the chicken on both sides and continue to cook until barely done, about 4 to 5 minutes. Transfer to serving plates. Keep warm in a 200° F oven where they will continue to lightly cook.
2. Using the same pan, melt 1 teaspoon margarine over medium heat. Add the onion and sauté for 2 minutes or until translucent. Add the mushrooms and sauté for 2 minutes. Turning the heat to high, add the broth and deglaze while constantly scraping the bottom of the pan. Reduce the broth by half, about ⅛ cup, about 1 minute. Add the bourbon and reduce until the alcohol has evaporated, about 1 minute. Turn the heat to low, add the cornstarch mixture, if using, and stir to thicken. Remove from the heat, and season to taste. Spoon over the chicken breasts.

Turkey Salad with Raisins M

Yield: 2 servings

This easy-to-make salad is high in protein, phosphorus, potassium, niacin (vitamin B_3), and the amino acids leucine, glutamic acid, and lysine. Using Soybean Mayonnaise as a creamy dressing, this delicious salad is egg-free.

*2 cups (10 ounces) cooked
  1-inch-cubed turkey
  or chicken*
3/4 cup diced celery
*2 to 3 tablespoons
  chopped scallion*
1/2 cup raisins
*1 teaspoon fresh lemon,
  lime, or grapefruit
  juice*

*Freshly ground white
  pepper to taste*
*1/3 cup Soybean Mayon-
  naise (page 188)*
*Spinach or Swiss chard
  leaves*

1. Mix all ingredients except spinach or Swiss chard leaves.
2. Mound on the spinach or Swiss chard leaves and serve.

Turkey Hash M

Yield: 2 servings

It is unfortunate that the word *hash* so often conjures up memories of dreary chopped meat and potatoes, for with just a modicum of care this simple and homey dish can be transformed into a sophisticated and delectable one. Turkey Hash is not only high in essential amino acids and minerals and low in fats but also a great way to use up leftover holiday turkey.

1½ teaspoons dairy-free, low-fat margarine
1 teaspoon oat, wheat, or rye flour
⅛ cup chopped onion
1 cup (6 ounces) diced steamed or baked potatoes
2 tablespoons chopped fresh parsley

½ teaspoon fresh thyme or sage or ⅛ teaspoon dried
1¼ cups (8 ounces) cubed cooked turkey
⅓ cup turkey broth
Freshly ground white pepper and nutmeg to taste

1. Heat a medium nonstick sauté pan until warm and melt the margarine. Over medium heat sprinkle in the flour and make a "Creole" roux by constantly stirring the flour until it turns medium brown and is fragrant, about 3 to 4 minutes.

2. Over low heat, add the onion and sauté for 2 minutes or until barely translucent. Add the potatoes and sauté for 4 to 5 minutes. Add the parsley and thyme or sage and mix.

3. Over medium heat add the turkey and sauté for 2

minutes. Turn the heat to high. Deglaze the pan by pouring in the broth and vigorously scraping it with a wooden spatula to release all caramelized juices. Season to taste with the pepper and nutmeg. Heat for 1 to 2 minutes and the sauce will thicken. Serve immediately.

VARIATION: Substitute cooked chicken (use chicken broth) or roast beef (use beef broth) for the turkey in the same amounts.

Roasted Rock Cornish Game Hens with Red Grapes and Sage M

Yield: 2 servings

Rock Cornish game hens are wonderful for dinner parties or just as a treat for yourself—a dish that is a delight to the palate as well as the waistline. These hens can be prepared and cooked in less than an hour. The grapes and sage provide a marvelous contrast to the flavor of the roasted meat. Serve them with Braised Escarole (see page 159) and boiled brown rice or pearl barley.

2 Rock Cornish game   *2 teaspoons fresh sage*
  hens (1 pound each)   *or ½ teaspoon dried*
1 slice garlic (optional)   *1 cup seedless red or*
                                 green grapes

1. Remove any extra fat deposits attached to the skin near the cavities. Rinse the hens under cold running water and drain. Pat dry.
2. If using the garlic slice, rub the cavities with it and discard. Using half the sage for each hen, rub it inside the cavity and leave it there. Fill each cavity with ½ cup grapes. Close each cavity with a trussing needle so the grapes do not fall out. Preheat the oven to 550° F.
3. Place the hens breast up on a roasting rack. Place the rack on a baking sheet. Place it in the center of the oven and quickly pour water in the baking sheet to ¼ inch deep, so that no rendered fat will smoke or burn. Reduce the heat to 500° F. Sear the hens for 20 minutes.
4. Using two wooden spatulas, turn the hens breast down and reduce the heat to 350° F. Roast for 25 to 35

minutes or until a thermometer inserted in the cavity registers 165° F. Remove from the oven and let rest for 10 to 15 minutes so the juices are redistributed. Remove the trussing needles and serve.

Baked Shrimp and Feta
with Fresh Basil and Tomatoes M

Yield: 2 servings

This shrimp casserole is a marvelous mix of flavors; the hint of lemon and basil in the light tomato sauce blends beautifully with the creamy fresh cheese. Serve this on a bed of brown rice or pearl barley and complement it with a watercress salad for a wonderful warm-weather meal.

6 ounces feta cheese
1½ teaspoons oil
⅓ cup chopped onion
1 tablespoon minced garlic
2 cups (1 pound) chopped seeded plum tomatoes
¼ cup chopped fresh parsley
2 tablespoons fresh basil or ¼ teaspoon dried

1 tablespoon chopped fresh marjoram or ¼ teaspoon dried
1 teaspoon fresh lemon zest or peel, finely julienned
Freshly ground allspice and black pepper to taste
1 pound large shelled, deveined, raw shrimp

1. Break the feta into 1-inch pieces and drain between sheets of absorbent toweling. Reserve.
2. Heat a small casserole until warm. Add the oil. Over medium heat, sauté the onion for 3 minutes, without browning, or until barely translucent. Add the garlic and sauté for 30 seconds, without browning, or until pungent.
3. Add the tomatoes, parsley, basil, marjoram, and lemon zest. Simmer over low heat for 10 minutes, stirring

occasionally. Season to taste. Remove from heat. The
sauce will look dry at this point; during baking the feta
and shrimp will release enough juice to make a light
sauce.

4. Preheat the oven to 400° F. Nestle the shrimp in the
sauce and sprinkle the feta on top. Bake for 12 to 15
minutes or until the shrimp are cooked.

Chinese Steamed Red Snapper M

Yield: 2 servings

The red snapper in this recipe is prepared in a manner common to many Chinese fish dishes—it is steamed until moist and flavorful and then topped with contrasting crunchy vegetables and a light sauce, which adds a distinctive finishing touch. If you have never steamed this fish before, you will find that the flavor is very delicate and sweet, unlike broiled, sautéed, or fried red snapper. One of the most popular quick dishes I teach in my cooking school, it is also a versatile dish that goes equally well with European and American menus.

1½ to 2 pounds whole red snapper, scaled and cleaned
1 teaspoon oil
2 tablespoons julienned bamboo shoots
¼ cup julienned green pepper and/or sweet red pepper
2⅔ tablespoons julienned scallions

2 teaspoons julienned fresh ginger root
½ cup (9 medium) dried Chinese black mushrooms, soaked in hot water and squeezed of excess water (optional), stems removed, or fresh mushrooms, julienned

Sauce

4½ tablespoons shao-hsing wine or dry sherry
3½ tablespoons light soy sauce or broth

(chicken or vegetable)
2⅓ tablespoons broth (chicken or vegetable)

1. Place a heat-resistant plate inside the steamer and bring water to full steam. Put the fish on the plate, cover, and steam for 12 to 15 minutes or until tender when pierced with a fork.
2. Heat a nonstick wok or sauté pan until hot and add the oil. Stir-fry the bamboo shoots, pepper, scallions, ginger, and mushrooms for 20 seconds. Reserve.
3. Heat the sauce ingredients in a small saucepan.
4. To serve, transfer the fish to a serving platter and sprinkle the stir-fried vegetables over it. Pour the warm sauce over all.

VARIATIONS: 1. Substitute julienned carrots, celery, fresh mushrooms, or zucchini for the other vegetables used in similar quantities.

2. Substitute striped bass, flounder, or petrale sole for the red snapper.

3. Fish filets may be substituted for whole fish. For 2 servings, steam 12 to 16 ounces of filets for 4 to 6 minutes per ½-inch thickness.

Tuna Niçoise M

Yield: 2 servings

Tuna Niçoise is a wonderful medley of textures, colors, and flavors. This healthful salad contains a good balance of protein, carbohydrate, and fat, and is high in vitamins A and C, potassium, calcium, phosphorus, and niacin (vitamin B_3). Ideal for warm weather, Tuna Niçoise is quick and easy to make and low in calories.

1 cup (6½-ounce can water-packed, low-sodium) tuna
¼ cup diced celery
¼ cup diced sweet red pepper
¼ cup diced kirby cucumber

1½ tablespoons thinly sliced scallion
1 tablespoon coarsely chopped fresh Italian parsley
Freshly ground black pepper to taste

Garnish (any or all optional)

Leaf lettuce
1 hard-boiled egg, quartered lengthwise
6 black olives (Niçoise,

ripe California, or Calamata)
1 sliced ripe tomato

1. Combine the tuna, celery, red pepper, cucumber, scallion, and parsley in a bowl and toss.
2. Season with black pepper to taste.
3. To serve, arrange the lettuce leaves on individual plates and mound the Tuna Niçoise on top. Place the quartered egg, olives, and tomato slices attractively on the plate.

VARIATION: Fresh tuna may be substituted for the canned. Purchase an 8-ounce tuna steak. Broil for 6 to 7 minutes, turn over and broil for 6 to 7 minutes more. Cool and break into flakes with a fork.

Papillotes E, R, M

Yield: 2 to 4 servings

Papillotes, a classic French dish, make a spectacular presentation. Wrapped in parchment paper or foil,* fish and vegetables steam in their own juices while being baked in the oven. This method enhances the flavor and tenderness. Extremely simple to make, Papillotes are ideal for quick, easy meals—and there are no pans to clean afterwards!

For Each Papillote

6 to 8 ounces fish (red snapper, pompano, bass, or sea scallops)

2 to 3 leaves Bibb lettuce or escarole

Vegetables (use a variety in small amounts)

1 leek, white part only, thinly sliced

2 fresh mushrooms, cleaned with stems removed

2 dried Chinese black mushrooms, soaked in hot water and squeezed of excess water, stems removed

¼ fennel bulb, cut into thin slices

1 endive, split lenghtwise into quarters

6 snow peas, strings removed

Freshly ground white pepper to taste

---

* For a special dinner party, use the parchment paper and for a quick meal, use the foil.

For Each Papillote

Parchment paper or
aluminum foil, 14 to
16 inches wide by 20 to
24 inches long
2 teaspoons grapeseed

or peanut oil (for
parchment paper only)
Straw for parchment
paper

Preparing the Papillote

Work on a completely dry surface.
1. Prepare the fish filet by removing all bones with a tweezers or your fingers, and patting it dry. Cut the parchment, rounding the corners to make an oval shape.
2. Make the Papillote up to 20 minutes before cooking. To begin, fold the paper or foil in half horizontally, and crease along the fold. Unfold. If using paper, rub oil over the entire insides. There should be a light layer of oil only, no large droplets of oil.

   Arrange the Bibb lettuce or escarole in the center of the paper or foil next to the fold line. Arrange the fish and vegetables on top of the lettuce or escarole. Season the fish and vegetables to taste with pepper.
3. At the fold line, fold the paper or foil over the fish and vegetables, making sure the ends meet. Beginning at one end of the cut edges next to the fold line, fold the edge over on itself. Fold this section over on itself again, pressing down so a tight seal is formed. Use either of the following tricks: If you want your Papillote to puff up like a balloon for an impressive presentation, if using foil, round the top layer of foil so it looks slightly puffed. Seal completely. If using paper, fold all of the edges except for the last inch. Insert the straw and wrap the paper around the straw so no air can escape. Blow into the center of the Papillote. The blowing will cause the paper to puff up. When the top of

the paper is rounded from the air trapped inside, remove the straw, making sure that no air escapes. Quickly
fold and seal this remaining edge. Press down firmly on
the folded edges once more as a final seal.

To Cook the Papillote

4. Heat the oven to 550° F with the baking sheet in the
oven. Open the oven door and slide the sheet out. Place
two Papillotes on the sheet, slide back into the oven,
and close the door. Maintain the heat at 500° F. The
heat will come in contact with the cold Papillote and
cause it to puff like a balloon. (If the Papillote does not
puff, the seal was not tight and air escaped. The ingredients will still be cooked and taste good; the Papillote
simply will not look as appealing and impressive.)
Cook the Papillote for 5 minutes for every ½-inch
thickness of fish filet.

To Serve the Papillote

5. Have everything ready for the presentation of the Papillote; it must be removed from the oven and served
immediately. Have a decorative pair of scissors at the
table ready for use.

Open the oven door and slide a large spatula under
the Papillote. Transfer it to the serving plate and serve
.. ..s is to the diner. Cut the top part of the paper and
fold it back. Let the diner eat from the interior of this
package.

If preferred, the paper can be opened in the kitchen
before serving and the fish and vegetables transferred to
a serving plate.

Broiled Beefsteak, Florentine Style M

Yield: 2 servings

Flank steak is one of the leanest cuts of beef and also one
of the most flavorful. In the style of Florence, it is marinated in black pepper to enhance its flavor. Lemon or lime
wedges are served on the side so the diner can squeeze
some fresh juice on top of the broiled steak as an accent.

*1 pound trimmed flank
    steak*
*1 teaspoon fresh
cracked black pepper,
divided*

*1 lemon or lime, cut
    into wedges (optional)*

1. Cut the flank steak into two portions. Press ½ teaspoon
   black pepper into the surface of each steak with the ball
   of your hand. Cover tightly and marinate at room temperature for 1 hour.
2. Place the broiler pan 4 inches from the heat source.
   Preheat the broiler. Broil the flank steak 3 to 4 minutes
   for rare, 5 to 6 minutes for medium, and 7 to 8 minutes
   for well done, turning the steaks over midway through
   the cooking.
3. Transfer steaks to individual serving plates; if using the
   lemon or lime wedges, arrange on each plate and serve.

Meat Loaf M

Yield: 2 to 4 servings

Meat loaf, the American version of French country pâté, is often treated, as a catch-all dish that is baked until it is dry and gray. In this recipe, however, meat loaf is treated with the respect it deserves. I've omitted the egg and bread crumbs found in most meat loaf recipes, and added chopped onion and green pepper for flavor and tenderness. Shape the meat loaf gently and baste it with broth to keep it tender. Meat loaf really becomes a savory meal if you bake it only until it is rare or medium. Serve with Braised Escarole (see page 159).

*1 pound ground lean
   chuck*
*2 tablespoons chopped
   red onion or 1
   tablespoon minced
   shallots*
*¾ teaspoon minced
   garlic*
*3 tablespoons chopped
   green pepper*
*1½ tablespoons tomato
   paste*
*2 teaspoons fresh thyme
   or ½ teaspoon dried*

*1 tablespoon chopped
   fresh basil or ½
   teaspoon dried*
*2 tablespoons chopped
   fresh parsley*
*Freshly ground black
   pepper to taste*
½ cup beef broth
*½ teaspoon starch
   (potato, arrowroot, or
   water chestnut) mixed
   with 1 teaspoon water
   (optional)*

1. Mix all ingredients except broth and starch. Cover tightly and refrigerate for 4 to 24 hours.
2. Preheat the oven to 475° F. Shape the beef mixture into

a loaf and put it into a loaf pan that is large enough for the hot air to surround the meat loaf. Do not pack the meat mixture tightly or it will be tough and hard.

3. Place the pan in center of oven, reduce the heat to 450° F, and bake for 15 minutes. Reduce heat to 350° F and bake for 5 to 10 minutes longer for rare; 15 to 20 minutes for medium; and 30 minutes for well-done. Baste occasionally with the beef broth.

4. Remove the pan from the oven and transfer the meat loaf to a serving platter. If thickening the broth, pour it into a small saucepan. Over low to medium heat pour in the starch mixture while stirring. Serve beside the meat loaf in a separate bowl.

Stir-Fried Beef with Broccoli and Mushrooms M

Yield: 2 servings

This one-dish Cantonese recipe takes less than 10 minutes to cook.

1½ teaspoons minced
  ginger
1½ teaspoons minced
  garlic
3 tablespoons thinly
  sliced scallions
1 tablespoon Chinese
  light soy sauce
1 tablespoon shao-hsing
  wine or dry sherry
2 teaspoons oil, divided
10 ounces flank steak,
  sliced ⅛ inch thick
2 cups broccoli flower-
  ets, split into 1½-inch-dia-
  meter pieces
½ cup (10) dried
  Chinese black mush-
  rooms, soaked in hot
  water and squeezed of
  excess water, stems

removed, or fresh
  mushrooms
½ cup ¼-inch slices of
  onion
2 teaspoons Chinese red
  vinegar or cider
  vinegar
⅓ cup beef broth
2 tablespoons oyster
  sauce (optional)
⅛ teaspoon freshly
  ground white pepper
1½ teaspoons sesame oil
  (Japanese or other
  Asian)
½ teaspoon starch
  (water chestnut, ar-
  rowroot, or potato)
  mixed with 1 table-
  spoon water

1. Combine the ginger, garlic, and scallions, and reserve.
   Combine the soy sauce and shao-hsing wine or sherry,
   and reserve.

2. Heat a nonstick wok or sauté pan until hot over high heat. Pour in 1 teaspoon oil. Over high heat, stir-fry the beef just until it loses its pink appearance, not more than 1 minute. Quickly remove and reserve in a bowl.

3. Pour in the remaining teaspoon oil. Over high heat, stir-fry the broccoli for 2 to 3 minutes or until almost tender. Add the mushrooms and stir-fry for 30 seconds. Add the onion and stir-fry for 30 seconds. Add the ginger, garlic, and scallions and stir-fry for 10 seconds.

4. Pour the soy sauce and shao-hsing wine or sherry around the sides of the wok or pan. Do the same with the vinegar. Add the broth and simmer for 1 minute. Add the beef, nestle in the broth, and simmer for 30 seconds. If using, add the oyster sauce and mix. Add the pepper and sesame oil and mix. Thicken with the starch mixture and serve immediately on a bed of rice or rice noodles.

Veal Pojarski E, R, M

Yield: 2 servings

Veal Pojarski is a classic dish consisting of ground meat flavored with onion, herbs, and spices. It is also one of the most versatile because of the variety of ingredients that can be used to change the flavor and character. Pojarski can be mixed up to one day in advance of cooking, and it takes less than 20 minutes to cook, which makes it great for entertaining.

1 pound ground raw veal
¼ teaspoon minced garlic
1 tablespoon finely chopped onion or scallion
1 teaspoon fresh thyme or ⅓ teaspoon dried
Freshly ground allspice and white pepper to taste

1 cup broth (chicken, veal, or vegetable), divided
¼ teaspoon starch (potato, arrowroot, or water chestnut) mixed with 1 tablespoon broth (optional)

1. Mix the veal, garlic, onion or scallion, herb and spices together. Refrigerate tightly covered for 2 to 24 hours. (The longer this mixture marinates, the fuller and more uniform its flavor will be.)
2. Shape the mixture into 2 or 4 oval-shaped patties. Heat a small nonstick sauté pan. Add ⅓ cup broth and heat. Place the patties in the pan and lightly sear on both sides, about 2 minutes per side.
3. Turn the heat to high. Pour in the ⅔ cup broth to deglaze the pan while constantly scraping the bottom of the pan

to release any caramelized juices. Turn the heat to low and simmer, partially covered, for 3 minutes (4 patties) or 5 minutes (2 patties). Turn the patties over and simmer again for the same time. Transfer the patties to serving plates.

4. If desired, pour in the starch mixture to thicken the sauce while constantly scraping the bottom of the pan. The sauce will turn glossy and thicken in a few seconds. Pour the sauce over the Veal Pojarski and serve.

VARIATION: To make *Chicken Pojarski*, an excellent variation, substitute 1 pound ground raw chicken for the veal. Marjoram is also delicious with this mixture; allow 1 teaspoon fresh marjoram (or ¼ teaspoon dried) and substitute nutmeg for the allspice.

Spaghetti with Bolognese Sauce R, M

Yield: 4 servings

When I was little, my favorite dish was Bolognese sauce, or spaghetti as it was known in the Midwest. Today I indulge in a modified version of this beloved dish. Here is my recipe, a good balance of protein, fat, and carbohydrate. It's rich and savory, and if you don't eat it all yourself, it's bound to go easy on your waistline.

1 teaspoon oil
½ cup chopped onion or leek
½ cup diced celery
½ cup diced carrot
2 teaspoons minced garlic
8 ounces ground lean fresh round steak
8 ounces ground fresh veal
1¼ cups broth (veal, beef, or vegetable)
1 tablespoon chopped fresh parsley
1 small dried bay leaf

2 teaspoons fresh oregano or ½ teaspoon dried
1½ tablespoons fresh basil or ¾ teaspoon dried
⅛ teaspoon fresh ground nutmeg
4 cups (2 pounds) chopped plum tomatoes
½ cup (6 ounces) tomato paste
Freshly ground black pepper to taste

Garnish (optional)

Freshly grated Parmigiano-Reggiano (cow's milk), Asiago (cow's milk), or

Pecorino Romano (sheep's milk) cheese to taste

1. Heat a nonstick casserole or sauté pan until warm and add the oil. Over medium heat sauté the onion or leek, celery, and carrot for 2 minutes. Add the garlic and sauté for 1 minute without burning it. Add the beef and veal and sauté until both lose their pink color, about 5 minutes.

2. Pour in the broth and add the parsley, bay leaf, oregano, basil, nutmeg, tomatoes, and tomato paste. Simmer over low heat for 2 to 2½ hours. Season to taste with pepper. If the sauce gets too dry, pour in some extra broth or water. Serve immediately over warm fettuccine or spaghetti and sprinkle with freshly grated cheese. This sauce can be refrigerated for up to 2 days. Warm over low heat for 15 minutes before serving.

Linguine with 30-Minute Fresh Tomato Sauce R, M

Yield: 2 servings

To ensure that this easy-to-make sauce has a bright, fresh taste, select only ripe plum tomatoes, because they are meaty and intensely flavored compared to other varieties. If you use tomato paste, be sure to use it sparingly or the light, fresh flavor will be obliterated by a strong canned taste. For a subtle and delicious accent, add a little bit of the same wine you are serving with the meal to the sauce. Serve on top of a bowl of steaming linguine, and top with freshly grated cheese.

2 teaspoons oil
¼ cup chopped red onion
2 teaspoons minced garlic
1¾ cups (14 ounces) chopped ripe plum tomatoes
2 to 4 tablespoons tomato paste
2 tablespoons chopped fresh parsley

1½ tablespoons chopped fresh basil or ¾ teaspoon dried
2 teaspoons fresh oregano or ½ teaspoon dried
Freshly ground black pepper to taste
6 tablespoons red wine (optional)

Garnish (optional)

Freshly grated Parmigiano-Reggiano (cow's milk), Asiago (cow's milk), or

Pecorino Romano (sheep's milk) cheese to taste

Heat a nonstick sauté pan, add the oil, and sauté the onion for 3 minutes over low heat. Add the garlic and sauté for 1 minute. Add the tomatoes, tomato paste, parsley, basil, oregano, and pepper to taste and simmer over low heat for 20 minutes. If using the wine, stir it in. Continue to simmer for 6 minutes. Serve on top of linguine and sprinkle with freshly grated cheese.

Shish Kebabs M

Yield: 2 servings

Shish kebabs are festive yet so easy that they can appear regularly on your menus. They are a great fix-your-own dish, and children, in particular, have loads of fun making them. Little preparation is involved, there is virtually no cleanup, and everyone dines on what he or she likes.

*1 pound trimmed leg of
   lamb, cut into 1½-inch
   cubes*

Marinade

*2 tablespoons chopped
   onion*
*1 small garlic clove,
   pressed*
*1 tablespoon fresh
   marjoram or 1
   teaspoon dried*

*1½ teaspoon fresh
   oregano or ½ tea-
   spoon dried*
*2 tablespoons fresh
   lemon or lime juice*
1 teaspoon oil

Vegetables

4 medium fresh mushrooms
*1 small green pepper,
   cut into ½-inch strips*
*4 plum tomatoes, cut
   into ¾-inch-thick
   slices*

*8 small red-skinned new
   potatoes, steamed,
   split in half*
*1 small zucchini, cut
   into ½-inch-thick
   discs*

6 metal skewers

1. Place the lamb in a bowl and add the marinade. Mix well. Cover tightly and chill for 24 hours so the meat will absorb some of the marinade's flavors. Stir once to distribute flavors uniformly. (While the marinade's flavor may seem assertive, remember that the meat is so dense that it will only be mildly enhanced by it.)

2. Remove meat from refrigerator 30 minutes before cooking. Prepare the vegetables. Adjust the rack so the shish kebabs will be 4 inches from the heat source. Preheat the broiler or grill.

3. Skewer the meat and vegetables loosely so all surfaces will get cooked. Alternate the ingredients, beginning and ending with the pepper strips.

4. Broil or grill the shish kebabs 9 minutes for rare, 12 minutes for medium, and 15 minutes for well-done meat.

Lamb Keftah M

Yield: 2 servings

Keftah is ground lamb or beef delicately seasoned with mint and spices. It is shaped into either kebabs or meatballs and then broiled. For a delicious Middle Eastern dinner that is well balanced, serve Keftah with Vegetable Rice Salad (see page 154).

*12 ounces ground lean
    raw lamb or chuck*
*2 tablespoons millet
    meal or coarsely
    ground oats moistened
    with 2 teaspoons
    water*
*3 tablespoons finely
    chopped onion, scal-
    lion, or shallot*
*2 tablespoons finely
    chopped parsley
    (optional)*
*½ teaspoon minced
    garlic*

2 teaspoons oil
*1½ teaspoons minced
    fresh mint leaves or
    ¾ teaspoon crumbled
    dried*
*⅛ teaspoon ground
    cinnamon (optional)*
*⅛ teaspoon ground
    allspice*
*⅛ teaspoon freshly
    ground black pepper*

1. Combine all ingredients and refrigerate for 2 to 24 hours so the flavors blend.
2. Shape into 6 3-inch-diameter meatballs or 6 1½-inch-diameter kebabs.
3. To broil, place the broiler pan 4 inches from the heat source. Brown the kebabs or meatballs on all sides.

   The cooking time for the meatballs will be 4 to 5 minutes for rare; 6 to 7 minutes for medium; 8 to 9 minute for well-done. Reduce the cooking time for the kebabs by 1 to 2 minutes.

Desserts

All of the recipes in the Dessert section are corn-free, wheat-free, cow's milk-free, cane sugar-free, soy-free, and egg-free. All are baker's and brewer's yeast-free except for the Baked Apples if date sugar is used.

Pineapple Mousse Sorbet E, R, M

Yield: 4 servings

Freezing pureed pineapple transforms it into a light, airy mousse. In this sorbet the luscious flavor and natural sweetness of this tropical fruit is highlighted without the addition of any sugar.

½ ripe pineapple (2 cups)
   or 2 cups unsweetened
   canned pineapple with
   juice

Trim the pineapple and cut it into small cubes. Puree in a blender or food processor (using the steel chopping blade).

Making the Sorbet

If using an ice-cream machine, freeze according to manufacturer's instructions. Serve immediately.

To freeze *without* an ice cream machine: Place the pineapple mixture in a metal cake pan, 9 × 9 inches, and freeze. Make sure the pan is placed evenly on the coldest surface of the freezer. Freeze for 45 to 60 minutes, stirring occasionally to distribute cyrstals evenly. Serve immediately.

Grapefruit Sorbet E, R, M

Yield: 4 servings

The light citrus flavor of pink grapefruit combined with the pungency of cloves makes a refreshing end to a meal. This sorbet can also be used as an intermezzo in a meal to clear the palate. One of the most popular desserts taught in my cooking school, it is very high in vitamin C and low in calories.

*2 cups freshly squeezed
pink grapefruit juice
(3 medium-size grape-
fruit)*

*2 to 3 tablespoons
honey mixed with 1
tablespoon water
Pinch ground cloves*

Making the Sorbet

If using an ice-cream machine: Mix the grapefruit juice and honey syrup. Add cloves to taste. Freeze according to manufacturer's instructions. Serve immediately.

To freeze *without* using an ice-cream machine: Mix the grapefruit juice and honey syrup. Add ground cloves to taste. Place the juice mixture in a metal cake pan, 9 × 9 inches, and freeze. Make sure the pan is placed evenly on the coldest surface of the freezer. Freeze for 45 to 60 minutes, stirring occasionally to distribute crystals evenly. Serve immediately.

Serving the Sorbet

Scoop sorbet into champagne flutes or coupes or large red wine goblets.

Strawberries Cardinal M

Yield: 4 servings

As the trend for fresh and light dining continues, fruit desserts are gaining in popularity. Instead of offering guests just a bowl of berries, try this update of Strawberries Cardinal, a classic French dessert.

*1⅓ cups (1 pint) sliced
    strawberries*
*⅓ cup freshly squeezed
    orange juice*

*½ cup (4 ounces)
    raspberries*

1. Marinate the strawberries in orange juice for 1 to 4 hours.
2. Puree the raspberries in a blender or food processor (using the steel chopping blade). Press through a sieve or colander to remove the seeds.
3. To serve, drain the strawberries, place in compotes or wineglasses and top with raspberry sauce.

Baked Apples E, R, M

Yield: 2 servings

This classic dessert is given a fresh new flavor by filling the apples with either pure maple syrup or date sugar and spices.

2 apples	*Ground cinnamon,*
1 tablespoon pure maple	*cloves, and nutmeg to*
syrup or date sugar	*taste*

1. Remove the stem and the top two-thirds of the core. Fill with the syrup or sugar, and spices if desired. Preheat the oven to 375° F.
2. Line a pie plate with aluminum foil. Place the apples, flat, on the plate. Place the plate in the center of the oven, reduce the heat to 350° F, and bake for 15 to 20 minutes or until just tender when pierced with the sharp point of a knife. Serve while warm or at room temperature.

VARIATION: The following varieties of apples are equally good for this dessert: Rome, Cortland, Empire, Gravenstein, Northern Spy, or Spartan.

Chinese Steamed Pears, E, R, M

Yield: 2 servings

In this delicate, subtle dessert, the blending of fragrant spices emphasizes the natural sweetness of the pears. Steamed Pears make a fine ending to French or American dinners as well as Chinese.

2 ripe pears (Comice or Barlett)
⅛ teaspoon ground cinnamon

⅛ teaspoon ground nutmeg
1 tablespoon honey

1. Remove the top three-quarters of the core of the pear. This will leave a cavity to be seasoned with the spices and honey. To prevent the liquid from pouring out of the pear, do not remove the bottom section of the core.
2. Mix the cinnamon, nutmeg, and honey together. Fill each cavity with this mixture up to ½ inch from the top. Stand the pears up on a heat proof procelain plate.
3. Bring the water in a steamer to a boil. Place the plate of pears inside the steamer. Cover. Steam the pears for 5 to 10 minutes or until just tender. Remove and serve warm in individual bowls.

SECTION **III**

Rebuilding Your Immune System

CHAPTER TEN

Putting Your Immune Power to Work for You

CONGRATULATE YOURSELF—you've already made the commitment to spectacular immune health. The diet and recipes in the previous section are helping you to remove the common foods that can damage your immune system, and to lose weight in the process. That's the REMOVE aspect of the Immune Power Diet. The rest of this book works on the simultaneous REBUILD aspect. It will help you achieve a perfectly tuned, radically strengthened, immune system by REBUILDING your immune system defenses to provide strong, powerful immune health.

But before you go on, you need a way to measure how your immune system is right now. In order to make your immune system more powerful, you need an objective way to know where you are now, and a way to measure your progress as you go along.

HOW SMART IS YOUR IMMUNE SYSTEM?

That's where the IQ comes in. I'm not talking here about your Intelligence Quotient—what people usually mean by "IQ"—but an even more important kind of IQ: your Immune Quotient. (I say even *more* important because it doesn't matter how intelligent you are if you don't have the health and vitality to use and enjoy that intelligence.)

The Immune Quotient (IQ) is a new and remarkable way to determine the status of your immune health. It is based on your personal diet, exercise, stress, and life-style factors. It includes all the elements that can affect immune health to enable you to draw a composite picture of your immune status.

The Immune Quotient is concerned with both the components that *help* your immune cells and those factors such as masked food allergies and adverse aspects in your life-style (smoking, too much alcohol, an unhealthy work environment, etc.) that may be damaging your immune system.

In short, your Immune Quotient will give you a profile of the things you can control. This is an IQ that you can improve, demonstrably and dramatically. You can, in effect, make your immune system "smarter" by strengthening every aspect of it.

TAKING YOUR IQ

In the following chapters, you will find six short assessment quizzes. Answer each question as accurately as possible. I believe that if you conscientiously answer my IQ quizzes, which are based on the many factors that medical research has shown to affect your body's immune capacity, you will have a useful assessment of your current immune status. After you total your score for each quiz, transfer that score into the appropriate space on the IQ chart on pages 305–6. After you have taken all six quizzes, total all of your individual IQ scores to get your Comprehensive IQ.

Et voilà! Your Comprehensive IQ will determine exactly

which supplement plan *you* need to bring your immune system to its strongest, most powerful level possible; what balance of vitamins, minerals, and amino acids you need to develop the areas where your immune system is weakest. Your IQ places you in one of five levels. No IQ is "better" or "worse"; each merely indicates the particular program of supplements that will mobilize your immune power to its highest level.

YOUR IQ: A PERSONALIZED PROGRAM

My goal is not just to have you understand the specific roles that substances like zinc, vitamin E, linoleic acid, and tryptophan play in immune health. Any basic nutrition book can do that. What I will do is show you how these immunity-enhancers fit into *your* life. When you have determined your Comprehensive IQ, you can determine exactly what supplements and how much of each of them you need to rebuild a powerful, efficient immune system.

You'll be able to see your Immune Quotient improve as you follow my program. I have seen such changes in my patients who followed my Immune Power Diet recommendations. You, too, could see more, stronger fighter T cells, increased antibody response, and high levels of all the chemicals essential to a mighty immune defense.

The most important results won't happen under a microscope, but in your life—how you feel, look, and act. By the end of this program you can expect an extraordinarily wide range of improvements in every area of your health. Joint pains, headaches, skin disorders, and stomach problems may be reduced, as may fatigue, depression, and insomnia.

MORE IS NOT NECESSARILY BETTER

Why bother with an individualized assessment such as the IQ? If these supplements are immune enhancers, doesn't it make sense to give everybody as much of them as possible? Most emphatically not! Research shows that many of these substances produce the very best possible immune health only within a very specific dosage range. Massive doses can put a person well beyond that optical immune-health range. If your body contains enough of a given substance, even an average dose could put you over the top so that there would be less benefit for your immune system than if you had taken nothing at all!

Overdosing with certain crucial nutrients can also create a deficit of complementary nutrients. If the body's equilibrium is disturbed in this way, a wide range of toxic responses may follow. In view of the increasing use of self-prescribed supplements, many experts are concerned about indiscriminate nutrient overdose.

Even if we don't suffer specific toxic reactions, there are many nutrients—iron, zinc, and B vitamins are the best examples—that work best in a very narrow range. With these, too much is as destructive as too little, and ignorant self-dosing destroys the precise balance the immune system needs, leading as further away from the optimal immune health we want to achieve.

IMMUNE NUTRIENTS: WHERE ARE THE FACTS?

It would seem simple to look up the proper doses of these supplements and recommend them to everyone, right?

Well, it's surprisingly hard to find out just how much *is* enough. Any physician has access to information about all prescription drugs and their proper dosage, method of administration, benefits, effects, and risks. There are reams of information available on drugs that are highly toxic, very specialized, or used only rarely. Yet there is shockingly little information about something as simple as vitamin and mineral supplements.

Sadly, we know more about how esoteric drugs with unpronounceable names affect a rat's liver than we do about how some vitamins work in people. During my years in medical school and practice, as well as when I was engaged in the research needed for this book, I made exhaustive literature and computer searches for this information. I am constantly amazed at how little relative attention has been paid to the way these natural supplements work to improve our immune health. In a country as medically advanced as ours, it is shocking that there is so little information about basic nutrient levels, and such a dearth of carefully controlled research.

Happily, recent years have produced breakthrough research in the field that is illuminating uncharted areas. Authorities estimate that new findings in this most revolutionary science are doubling every four years. That is an amazing statement: *fully half* of what we now know about immune-enhancing substances was discovered in the last four years; and in four years from now, we should know *twice as much*. Physicians, public health scientists, epidemiologists, and biostatisticians have begun to study the effect of nutrient supplements in large numbers of people over long periods. The scientific community is starting to realize that the entire area of immuno-nutrition carries the single best hope of radically changing our idea of health by our learning to *prevent* diseases and suffering.

The Federal government gave a boost to this research when scientists at the Food and Drug Administration created a standard known as the Minimum Daily Requirement (MDR), which indicates levels of vitamins and minerals adequate for health.

In fact, the MDR measures only the absolute *lowest* level of each nutrient necessary to avoid becoming seriously, actively sick. Granted, if you follow these recommendations, you won't get deficiency diseases like scurvy (caused by a lack of vitamin C) or pellagra (due to a lack of niacin). But, in fact, these standards are inadequate for true immune power.

We need much *higher* levels of several nutrients to maximize our health and feel truly alive and vigorous. This is especially true if your IQ is significantly low, for that means your immune system has been chronically undernourished. You have learned to live with this and the subtle (and not so subtle) effects of long-term deficits; you will need bold, aggressive treatment to make up for those long-term imbalances.

If you are familiar with the Minimum Daily Requirement, you will notice that my recommended doses are clearly much larger. My experience has convinced me that these are much more realistic, practical doses to repair, rebuild, and renew a tired immune system.

The program I outline in chapter 14 is based on exactly these rebuilding principles. Whatever your IQ category, each plan is designed to actively rebuild your immune defenses.

Those are the principles which have given my patients such tremendous improvements in their health, weight, and vitality. Many of my patients found it hard to believe that they would feel such sweeping improvements in their lives. That's understandable, for after all, our immune system affects so much of our health, and the improvements are so dramatic, that even the most sober recitation of facts sounds like wild exaggeration.

But once my patients have followed my recommendations and discovered how terrifically strong and vital they feel, they can't believe they ever lived any other way.

In the next three chapters you'll find a wealth of very specific information on how you can rebuild your immune system to boost your Immune Quotient. This is the final step towards achieving superb "immune tune."

CHAPTER ELEVEN

Your Immune Vitamins

SECTION II showed you how to eliminate your danger foods and the immune damage they cause. But, that's only part of the Immune Power Diet program. The next few chapters will show you how to use this solid immune foundation to rebuild positive immune health.

THE POWER OF POSITIVE IMMUNE THINKING

Other scientists have recognized food sensitivities and their effects on the immune system. But, as incredible as it sounds, no one has taken the next logical, obvious step—adding a specifically tailored program to give the immune system the particular building blocks it needs to thrive.

Now, you will learn how to develop a carefully balanced supplementation plan with the vitamins, minerals, and amino acids necessary to rebuild and strengthen your immune system. With it, you can make sure your body has the specific nutrients it needs to keep producing the immune protectors—the lymphocytes and antibodies—you need.

In this and the following chapters, I want to give you a look at the scientific research findings that have helped me create the Immune Power Diet. These new scientific developments provide the strong scientific principles that make the Immune Power Diet succeed.

SHARPEN YOUR PENCILS

But first, I want to turn this chapter over to you, so you can check your vitamin readiness. This is the first Immune Quotient assessment quiz—your vitamin IQ. You can use it to get an overview of your vitamin status to determine where you have enough, and where you need to strengthen your vitamin intake.

THE VITAMIN IQ QUIZ

Circle a number for each question. At the end of the quiz, add the numbers to get your total Vitamin IQ. Then, transfer that score to the space marked "Vitamin IQ" on page 305. When you have taken all six IQ quizzes, you can add up the scores to get your Comprehensive Immune Quotient.

1. **During the past year, how often have you had a cold, flu, or other minor infectious illness?**
   5 Not at all
   4 Once
   3 2 to 3 times
   2 4 to 5 times
   1 More than five times

2. **Do you drink alcoholic beverages?**
   5 No
   4 Yes, less than one drink each day
   3 Yes, about two drinks a day, or several drinks about once per week
   2 Yes, several drinks on more than one occasion per week
   1 Yes, several drinks a day

3. **What is the condition of your skin?**
   5 Always healthy, good complexion
   4 Minor problems in the past, but healthy now
   3 Occasional skin problems
   2 Frequent skin problems
   1 Chronic, severe problems

4. **Do you take oral contraceptives?** *(For women only)*
   5 No
   4 Not now, but I have within the last six months
   3 Yes
   2 Yes, and I also drink alcohol occasionally
   1 Yes, and I also drink alcohol and smoke cigarettes

5. **How is your appetite?**
   5 Excellent, and it has always been fine
   4 It is usually good
   3 It is worse now than in the past
   2 Food doesn't taste good to me anymore
   1 I have to force myself to eat

6. **Which of the following best describes your eating pattern?**
   5 Several small balanced meals and snacks; I avoid junk food
   4 Usually nutritional and balanced, but not always
   3 Often skip meals; not much variety in diet
   2 I eat more snacks than meals; don't worry about nutrition
   1 Frequent "pig-outs" and binges, tend to overeat

7. **How often do you eat raw fruits and vegetables?**
   5 At least once each day
   4 Often, but probably not every day
   3 Sometimes
   2 Not often
   1 Rarely or hardly ever

8. **How often do you eat in fast food restaurants?**
   5 Never
   4 Once a week or less
   3 Two to four times a week
   2 Nearly every day
   1 At least one meal every day

9. **When you get a cold, does it ever require medical attention?**
   5 No, never
   4 Once or twice, but not usually
   3 Sometimes
   1 Yes, this often happens

10. **In general, do you remember your dreams?**
    5 Almost always
    4 Often
    3 Sometimes
    2 Rarely
    1 Never

11. **Are you under frequent physical or athletic stress?**
    5 No
    3 Yes, but only moderate stress
    1 Yes, severe physical stress

12. **Do you bruise easily?**
    5 No, never
    4 Very infrequently
    3 Sometimes
    1 Often

13. **How is your health now compared to other years?**
    5 Consistently good as long as I can remember
    4 Better now than it used to be
    3 About the same, with occasional illnesses
    2 Clearly worse now than it used to be
    1 I've always had poor health

14. **Are your hands, arms, or legs numb or painful when you wake up?**
    5 No
    4 Once in a very great while
    3 From time to time
    2 Frequently
    1 Almost always

15. **Is your learning ability as sharp as it once was?**
    5 Yes, just as good or better
    4 Not quite as good
    2 Clearly not as good
    1 Facts often slip my mind and I have trouble concentrating

16. **Do you work under strong fluorescent lights?**
    5 Not often
    4 Sometimes
    3 Frequently
    1 Every day

17. **Do you spend a large portion of your day in front of a television or computer monitor?**
    5 No
    4 Sometimes
    3 Frequently
    1 Every day

18. **If you know it, what is your blood cholesterol level?**
    5 very low
    4 low to medium
    3 medium to high
    2 high
    1 extremely high

TOTAL VITAMIN IQ ——— (transfer to page 311)

WHAT YOU DON'T KNOW *CAN* HURT YOU

Why is this quiz necessary? Don't you probably already have all the vitamins you need? You may think that because you eat relatively well, or take multiple vitamins, that your vitamin bank accounts are plenty full. You couldn't be more wrong.

Every few years the Department of Health and Human Services and the U. S. Department of Agriculture survey the nutrition of average, bascially healthy, Americans. Each time, these studies show that *millions of us are suffering from alarming vitamin shortages*. The combined results of the most recent studies show that Americans lack vitamin A and C; B vitamins thiamine, pyridoxine, and riboflavin, as well as calcium, iron, and magnesium.

FROM THE LABORATORY . . .

Researchers at MIT who tested 120 patients selected at random from those admitted to hospitals across the country found that only 12 percent showed proper levels of all vitamins. Eighty-eight percent had at least one serious deficiency, and 59 percent were short of at least two critical nutrients. In the MIT researchers' own words:

These studies . . . lead to the inescapable conclusion that a single nutrient deficiency can result in profound impairment of specific immunologic processes—a concept that has not yet received widespread attention or general acceptance. This inattention may be having important clinical results, since the immunologic deficiencies may significantly alter disease course and/or therapeutic response.

WHERE ARE YOU ON THE PIE?

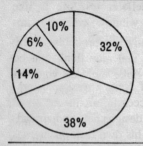

Incidence of Vitamin Deficiencies in U.S. Population

32%: one vitamin deficiency
38%: two vitamin deficiencies
14%: three vitamin deficiencies
6%: four vitamin deficiencies
10%: five vitamin deficiencies

I'm often asked, "But if I had a vitamin deficiency, wouldn't I know about it?" The answer is no: 60 percent of the people with deficiencies show no overt signs. You may well not feel anything really wrong because many of these symptoms are subtle and hard to pin down. Do you recognize any of these symptoms in yourself or your family?

WHAT HAPPENS WHEN YOU HAVE A VITAMIN DEFICIENCY?

Frequent colds and flu
Ear, eye, nose, or throat infections
Low energy
Swollen glands
Digestive problems
Blood disorders

Nervousness, sleep problems
Irritability

Poor concentration
Anxiety
Weight problems

You may feel just slightly below par—not quite as energetic, as healthy or as razor-sharp as you'd like, but you don't need to settle for second-rate health. You simply have no idea how spectacular you *can* feel, and what health, energy, and enjoyment you can tap by correcting vitamin deficiencies. With the deficiencies, life is like constantly looking through a dirty window, when by simply cleaning it, you can enjoy a sparkling, clear, unrestricted view.

Let me tell you about Edward, who was referred to me last fall by his physician, one of New York's most respected internists. Edward is a successful architect known for his highly innovative restaurant designs here and abroad. Only thirty-two years old, he runs his own firm of international architects, which requires a whirl of meetings, business trips, and an active social life. In early October, Edward had what seemed like the flu. He ran a slight fever, and was absolutely drained of energy. After a week in which he lost five pounds, he felt slightly better and decided he had to return to work. But even as he dragged himself into the office, he knew something was very wrong. This man, used to keeping fourteen-hour days, would awaken with barely enough energy to get out of bed, force himself through the morning's round of meetings, and then, at lunch, fall asleep. Alarmed, he went to his physician, who diagnosed a serious liver inflammation, acute viral hepatitis.

His doctor put it to him directly: there is nothing we can do for hepatitis except to wait until the body fights off the virus. A case of hepatitis as severe as his often means hospitalization for several weeks, and it was not uncommon for sufferers to be unable to work for several months. Edward knew that an absence that long could throw his whole company in jeopardy. His physician suggested he call me.

Although I had never treated a case like this, I knew Edward clearly needed a massive immune boost to help his body fight off the disease. I decided to follow the most basic rules of immune maintenance and prescribed a regime of vitamin supplements designed expressly to give his immune system massive reinforcement.

The Tuesday he began the vitamin treatment, Edward was bedridden, weak, and jaundiced, with high, intermittent fever. By Wednesday night, the fever and pain had dropped dramatically. The next day they were gone, and Edward was back in the office on Tuesday of the next week. Instead of suffering six to eight weeks, he returned to work in seven days, thanks to his immune-based vitamin therapy.

THE IMMUNE-POSITIVE VITAMINS

Vitamins are clearly among the most essential immune building blocks. We have long known that there are thirteen essential vitamins necessary for growth and health.

Each of these does a different job in your body. Do you find yourself more tired and fatigued than you feel you ought to be? People who say "yes" are often suffering from a lack of vitamin A, E, or C, or an imbalance of the B complex vitamins. Maybe you are plagued by nervous problems that make you seem tuned "too fast." Do you have trouble falling asleep? Are you often jittery, nervous, and anxious? Are you one of those people who seems to react much more strongly to financial, work, and family stresses than others? If you recognize yourself here, you can probably benefit by taking the "nerve tonic" vitamins: Pyridoxine (B_6), Niacin (B_3), and Cobalamin (B_{12}).

Mood and emotions can also reflect our vitamin levels. Do you often find yourself depressed or blue? Do you often explode irritably at those around you? Do you notice yourself riding a mood roller coaster, where you're happy, then gloomy, in the space of a few hours? If any of these sound familiar, your vitamin accounts may be out of balance. You might be a good candidate for the B vitamins, especially Thiamine (B_1) and Cobalamin (B_{12}).

In addition to building and strengthening the body's cells, vitamins work with enzymes to speed up chemical reactions in the body. This means that proper levels of vitamins work to give us a faster, more aggressive immune defense. Although all vitamins are important, four are especially critical for strong immune health: C, E, A, and B complex.

VITAMIN C: THE SUPREME IMMUNE VITAMIN

More research has been done on vitamin C than on any other vitamin. I have stacks of studies in my office library that make one point clear: beyond any doubt, vitamin C (*ascorbic acid*) has the strongest positive effects on our immune system.

Here are some questions you can use to estimate your vitamin C levels:

- How often do you get sick? Are you one of those people who seems to catch every little thing that comes along, every flu bug and every cold?
- Do you bruise easily, showing black and blue or brown bruise marks often on your legs and arms?
- When you cut yourself, does it seem to take a long time for the blood to stop?
- Do you often get nosebleeds?

You may recall in chapter 4 that you met the four key parts of your immune system: the thymus, lymphocytes (some of which become T cells), antibodies, and macrophages. Obviously, the stronger each of these components, the better your overall immune health. Let's look at how this one vitamin helps your key immune players.

VITAMIN C AND YOUR IMMUNE SYSTEM

Dr. M. P. Dieter reported in *The Proceedings of the Society of Experimental Biology and Medicine* that the more vitamin C is in the diet the greater the weight of vital immune system tissues like the thymus and lymph nodes, and the more efficiently the thymus works preparing T cells to fight germs.

According to the *American Journal of Clinical Nutrition*, an international research team headed by Dr. R. Anderson of the University of Pretoria, South Africa, showed that volunteers' immune cells reacted more strongly to challenge testing after they took vitamin C supplements. The vitamin seems to help those cells engulf and destroy bacterial invaders. The study concludes that the vitamin supports the entire T cell component of our immune system.

The research team led by biochemist Dr. W. Prinz of the University of Witwatersrand Medical School, in Johannesburg, proved that vitamin C helps the body produce a chemical that triggers antibody production.

Dr. Stephen Vallance of Birmingham Hospital in England found that vitamin C directly increases levels of all the major types of antibodies. At MIT, Drs. Robert Gross and Paul Newberne did an encyclopedic review of the literature and found uniformly that vitamin C stimulates the immune cells—the macrophages—that "eat" invading germs. They also cite studies showing that the vitamin strengthens our white blood cells' ability to kill invaders in the body.

INTERFERON

Dr. Benjamin Siegel, a research pathologist at the University of Oregon in Portland, found in experiments that vitamin C is not only "significantly increased . . . immune responses," but also raised the blood level of interferon, one of the body's most potent germ fighting chemicals.

In short, vitamin C aids every part of your immune system: it strengthens the integrity of all the immune cells, makes them work more efficiently, and maintains the whole range of necessary helper chemicals.

Dr. Linus Pauling, the eminent biochemist and two-time Nobel Prize winner, has long been known for his research showing that vitamin C helps cure and prevent the common cold. A recent study reported in the *American Journal of Clinical Nutrition* supports this, reporting that volunteers had 20 percent fewer cold symptoms when taking vitamin C, and that it prevented colds in a large number of subjects.

I have often seen this in my practice. Sally was a delightful, vivacious woman of about thirty-five who came to me last year. Her complaint was simple: she got sick all the time. Scarcely three weeks went by that she wasn't either coming down with a cold, in bed with one, or just recovering. For Sally, winter meant a steady progression of dreary, drippy, uncomfortable colds, throat infections, running nose and eyes. Summer was hardly any better.

"For a while I thought they came from Kenny," she

said, referring to the eager four-year-old who sat on her lap. "You know how kids are always bringing bugs home, but none of the other mothers I know have it this bad. I feel like I must be keeping Kleenex in business, Doctor," she joked. "Isn't there something I can do?" Her tests showed she was free of any hidden problems that would explain her symptoms, but she was often under a lot of pressure, which can deplete vitamin C. Clearly, she needed an immune power boost, so I prescribed a program high in vitamin C.

I wondered how it had worked for Sally, because she hadn't been back into my office since she started the program. Then, over a year later, I ran into her at a local restaurant. "Well, Doctor, I wish I could report that I haven't had a cold all year, but I can't." She grinned michievously. "I had one. Period. Considering that's about a dozen less than last year, I'd call your treatment a success!"

"E" FOR IMMUNE EXCELLENCE

Vitamin E is another vitamin that provides immune power. Like C, vitamin E directly helps all the components of the immune system. But in addition, it has an even more extraordinary benefit. It has been called the "youth vitamin."

You may remember that I mentioned something called *free radicals*. These molecules are thought to disrupt cell processes, destroy vital cell enzymes, and damage cell membranes, which leads to mutations and cell destruction.

In his landmark research, Dr. Denham Harman proposed that the cumulative effect of free radical damage is the root of aging—and of all the debilitating, difficult, diseases that often come with it. Right this minute, although you can't feel it, your body is building up levels of free radicals, and these cellular saboteurs are doing more and more damage to your cells. If that damage is serious enough, you may fall prey to degenerative diseases like diabetes, rheumatoid arthritis, or cardiovascular disease. Additionally, these chemicals are hurting every one of your trillion immune fighters, thus lowering your resistance and leaving you open to disease.

Vitamin E is one of the most potent known antidotes to free radicals, chemically deactivating them before they can destroy cells. This is why scientists believe that Vitamin E helps produce a stronger, more positive, immune response.

For a rough check of your own vitamin E status, here are some things to look for:

- What happens when you get a scratch, a burn or some other minor injury? Does it start mending right away, and disappear in two weeks or so? Or do you find sores lingering on, taking forever to heal?
- Do you have scars that never completely healed?

If you are this kind of a slow healer, you might very well benefit from vitamins E and C, the skin repair vitamins.

ARE "E" MEN "HE-MEN"?

Vitamin E helps keep men sexually healthy, active and strong, and it is particularly necessary for healthy testicles and hormone production. Studies also show it seems to increase fertility in both men and women. Vitamin E may also cause short-term rises in our sex drive. While few clear studies have been done on this, many of my male patients have told me that during the first two or three weeks they started taking vitamin E, their sex drive noticeably increased.

More than any other single vitamin, E has been associated with sexual health and activity. In women it has been shown to relive menopausal symptoms like headaches and hot flashes, and to have a role in regulating menstrual flow. For men, it also helps prevent and cure inflammation of the prostate, one of the primary sex glands.

- Vitamin E also has a direct effect on the immune system. Physicians at Cornell University have shown that vitamin E stimulates antibody production and makes the immune cells more able to react with invading germs.
- Recent findings from a prominent team of Japanese immunologists have discovered that vitamin E causes our T cells to react faster and more strongly.
- Microbiologists in Colorado have shown that vitamin E makes animals less prone to bacterial infection, and that it significantly increased resistance to disease. In one study, vitamin E produced a 40 percent stronger response to tetanus germs, and stimulated antibody production in mice.

VITAMIN A:
THE GRADE-A IMMUNE HELPER

Vitamin A shares many of the properties of vitamin E. Proper levels of this vitamin work effectively to "sponge up" free radicals before they can do severe cell damage. In that respect, it provides the same range of positive health effects as vitamin E.

WHAT DOES YOUR SKIN TELL YOU?

If you want to take stock of your vitamin A status, one of the best tools is a mirror. Take a close look at your skin. Is it dry, flaky? Does it just seem lifeless, without any real suppleness or elasticity? If these are problems for you, you may be one of the people who need vitamin A for crucial skin care. (Vitamins E and B complex may also help you.)

VITAMIN A: DO THE EYES HAVE IT?

Do you find it increasingly difficult to see when the light gets low? Have you often been driving at dusk or at night and been unable to make out shapes of other vehicles, or had trouble reading road signs? If "yes" is your answer to these questions, you may not have enough vitamin A. This vitamin is crucial to your night vision. However, too much vitamin A is as bad as too little, so be sure never to exceed the recommendations I give you in chapter 14.

Researchers have found that children with low vitamin A had abnormally low levels of T cells in their blood—too few of the immune-cell soldiers to fight their immune battles.

In addition, vitamin A can actually make each immune cell fight *harder*. One research group found that vitamin A added to immune cells in a test tube dramatically energized these cells by 50 to 100 percent. That's the equivalent of having each cell fight *twice* as hard.

THE B VITAMINS:
THE IMMUNE POWER FAMILY

You need this vitamin family—there are twelve B vitamins—to help your immune cells do their work of keeping you healthy, energetic, and slim.

Many of my patients find the B vitamins confusing. That's understandable, because their names are complicated: several of the B vitamins have two names, and several of them don't even have the word "vitamin" in their names. To set the record straight, here's the complete list:

B VITAMIN FAMILY TREE

Thiamine B_1	Folacin (Folic Acid, Folate)
Riboflavin B_2	Choline
Niacin B_3	Inositol
Pyridoxine B_6	Biotin
Pantothenic Acid	Para-aminobenzoic Acid (PABA)
Cobalamin B_{12}	Pangamic Acid B_{15}

Although each of these vitamins has its own individual benefit, they really work as a team, and in order to work effectively, they have to be in the right balance and relation to one another. For that reason, they are often termed the "B complex" vitamins.

Doctors have begun to report truly astounding results of B vitamin therapy. One of my most dramatic successes was with a young man of twenty-six named Kirk, whose hair was already quite gray. Since childhood, Kirk had had a long history of severe behavior problems and had bounced in and out of mental hospitals, clinics and treatment facilities. He couldn't keep a job. He was alcoholic, and had chronic insomnia. His problems were so severe that even his own mother described her son as "impossible to live with."

I put him on a regimen that included large doses of the B vitamin pryidoxine, and in just three months he was able to sleep through the night. Soon, his mood and behavior improved dramatically. It was as though another person had been imprisoned inside him all those years, for his erratic, aggressive manner turned friendly and warm. He was able to get, and keep, a full-time job and soon stopped his alcohol abuse. And, to top off this believe-it-or-not story, his prematurely graying hair turned chestnut brown again. At last report, Kirk is living back home with his mother who says that "He's become a joy to love with!"

The B vitamins have equally dramatic effects in every area of your immune system. There is so much research that I have distilled it into a simple chart. Here are the ways that essential B vitamins help all of your immune defenders, and here is what happens when you don't have enough of them.

WHAT HAPPENS WHEN YOU HAVE A VITAMIN B DEFICIENCY?

Without Enough . . .	Immune System Problems
Thiamine B_1	Lower antibody response
	Thymus gland shrinks
Riboflavin B_2	Lower antibody response
Pyridoxine B_6	Lower antibody response
	Severe loss of T cells
	Less active immune cells
	Immune-producing tissues damaged
	Thymus gland shrinks
	Cell defense cycle interrupted

Without Enough . . .	Immune System Problems
Folacin (Folic Acid)	Immune-producing tissues damaged
	Fewer immune cells produced
	Lower immune cell defenses
Pantothenic Acid	Cell reaction cycle interrupted
	Lower antibody response
	Immune cell function disrupted
Biotin	Lower primary antibody response
	Lower secondary antibody response
Cobalamin B_{12}	Immune-creating tissues damaged
	Fewer immune cells produced
	Weaker bacterial killing

Before leaving the subject of the immune-crucial B vitamins, let's look at just a few of the most interesting research dispatches now coming in on vitamin B_6, one of the most essential of these B vitamins.

Pyridoxine (B_6) is the best studied of the B vitamins for its wide effects of our immune cells. Researchers have repeatedly found that without enough of this B vitamin, your immune tissues can actually shrink. The thymus and spleen, two of your most crucial immune organs, need pyridoxine for normal activity. In addition, pyridoxine deficiency was associated with fewer immune cells in the lymph nodes.

B₆ AND WATER BUILD UP

Look around your ankles, wrists, neck, and thighs—do you have puffy water build up? This problem, called *edema*, occurs when your body stores too much water in its tissues. Many women experience this extra fluid retention just before their menstrual period. Vitamin B₆ (Pyridoxine) can help.

If you have a real problem with edema, you may need to increase your vitamin B₆ (Pyridoxine). In correct doses, this works like a natural, safe diuretic, helping the body flush out extra water.

TAKING YOUR B'S THE RIGHT WAY

If you take any of the B vitamins, here are two things to remember:

- Pyridoxine (vitamin B₆) is a diuretic, and may make you need to urinate often. It's *not* a good idea to take this vitamin before you go to sleep; instead, take it in the morning or afternoon.
- Other B vitamins can make it hard to fall asleep. As a safe rule, you should take only B vitamins in the morning.

Cobalamin (B₁₂) was studied by Dr. Sandra Kaplan, who examined several patients suffering from vitamin B₁₂ deficiency. In the laboratory, she exposed their immune cells to a common bacteria and found that the immune cells' ability to destroy the bacteria was *more than one-third weaker* than cells from control patients with no B₁₂ deficiency.

Folic acid was studied by Dr. Robert Gross at MIT, who looked at the immune responses of twenty-three patients with folic acid deficiency. He found that these patients couldn't mount an effective immune response when challenged. However, when the patients were given folic acid supplements, their weakened immune responses returned to normal.

TOO MUCH OF A GOOD THING

Let's forget the laboratory for a moment, and talk about people. What does all this scientific evidence mean for *you?* Knowing all of this, doesn't it make sense to go out and take as many vitamins as possible? Emphatically not. Unlike money or friends, *more* vitamins are definitely not always better. Every vitamin works best within a certain dosage range, and taking too much can be as bad, or worse, than taking too little.

This is especially true with the fat-soluble vitamins—A, D, E, and K. Because these vitamins are stored in fat and not in watery tissues, the body can't flush them out when it has too much. If you're taking too much, you can suffer a wide range of symptoms: blurred vision, tremors, restlessness, kidney stones, ulcers, upset stomach, hair loss, nausea, rapid heartbeat, and high blood pressure.

What most people don't know is that even the water-soluble vitamins—vitamin C and the B complex vitamins—work best in certain amounts. A recent paper from the Mayo Clinic reported that several people who were taking megadoses of Pyridoxine (B_6) without medical supervision showed signs of serious overdose, including tingling and numbness in their hands and feet, unsteadiness, and lack of muscle coordination. Fortunately, this story ends happily: all of the patients reported their symptoms disappeared when they stopped overdosing themselves.

Another study, from India, showed that volunteers taking vitamin C boosted their immune strength—up to a point. But if they took too much, their cells were actually *less able* to kill bacteria, which shows a dramatic drop in immune strength. In another study, researchers in California found that high concentrations of vitamin C actually reduce immune cells' ability to kill fungal invaders in the body. The same is true of vitamin E; in the right doses, it stimulates the immune system, but too much of it actually brings about a weaker, less active immune response in people.

That is why each of us must design our individual carefully calibrated vitamin program. The vitamins you need depend on your age, sex, diet, health, exercise, stress level, and a host of other life-style factors.

MAKE YOUR VITAMINS EASY TO SWALLOW

Some of my patients find it inconvenient to have to juggle so many vitamin and mineral pills. It can be a chore to remember, store, and even swallow, a whole arsenal of pills. And the more trouble it is, the less you will want to stick with the program. Here are three good tips I give my patients so they can build vitamins into their lives with the least amount of bother.

- Multi-vitamins combine several vitamins, and some minerals, into one, easy-to-take pill or capsule. You can probably find one that contains several of the vitamins you need. Don't worry if the doses vary slightly from my recommendations. As long as the formula contains vitamins in approximately the recommended *proportions*, they will work, and will make it easier to get the nutrients you need.

- You can buy a small pill holder at any drug store. Many patients find these are helpful to keep a day's supply of supplements in order. They sort their pills once, and then divide them into each compartment.

- Certain vitamins work best if taken at a specific time of day. Although vitamins C and E can be taken any time during the day or evening, vitamins A and D are most effective if taken in the morning, and vitamin B complex can be taken in the morning or early afternoon.

VITAMIN SHOPPERS' TIPS

- Read all vitamin labels carefully. Often, vitamins contain fillers like starch, yeast, sugar, or corn, which can create serious allergy problems. To prevent them, always make sure to buy hypo-allergenic vitamins.

- When buying any B vitamins or vitamin C, try to get them in a time-release form. Because these are water-soluble vitamins, it helps your body absorb them better.

CHAPTER TWELVE

Minerals: Building Blocks for Immune Power

MINERALS STRENGTHEN your cells and supply vital nourishment so that your trillion immune soldiers can do their job right. Minerals are vital material that supplies your immune troops, to keep them—and you—active, strong, and resilient.

All minerals are not created equal in terms of strengthening immune health. There is a special family of four *Immune Power* minerals that we all need to keep our immune cells happy: zinc, iron, copper, and selenium.

MINERALS YOU NEED

The essential minerals we need are divided into two categories: *bulk minerals*—those your body uses in large quantity, and *trace minerals*—minerals that your body uses only in minute amounts, or traces.

Bulk Minerals	Trace Minerals
Calcium	Copper
Magnesium	Zinc
Sodium	Iron
Potassium	Manganese
Sulfur	Chromium
	Selenium
	Lithium
	Rubidium

To find out how you are doing in the mineral department, take a moment to test your mineral immune quotient.

THE MINERAL IQ QUIZ

---

1. **Overall, how satisfied are you with your sexual vitality?**
   5 Very satisfied
   4 Usually satisifed, but not always
   3 Neither satisfied nor dissatisfied
   2 Dissatisfied—I could use more sexual energy
   1 I have a significant problem with my sexual vitality

2. **How is your hair?**
   5 Healthy, full, and growing
   4 Mostly healthy, occasional minor dandruff or oiliness
   3 Dry, brittle or premature graying
   2 Very dry, lifeless
   1 I have a history of problem hair

3. **Do your fingernails have white spots on them?**
   5 I have never noticed it
   4 I have seen it, but rarely
   3 From time to time
   2 They do right now
   1 Usually or always

4. **How fast do your minor wounds, cuts, or burns heal?**
   5 Very fast, almost overnight
   4 Usually quickly, in a few days
   3 About average, a week or so
   2 Clearly more slowly than they used to
   1 Very slowly

5. How stable is your mood?

5 I am always very even tempered
4 I am usually even tempered
3 I notice I'm feeling more anxious or blue than I used to
2 I have real mood swings
1 I have real problems controlling my moods

6. Do you weigh more than you should?

5 No, and I never have
4 Not now, but I used to
3 My weight fluctuates a lot
2 I am currently overweight by more than five pounds
1 I have always had a weight problem

7. How many silver fillings do you have in your mouth?

5 None
4 1 to 2
3 3 to 4
2 More than 4

8. How many times a day do you drink coffee or caffeinated soft drinks?

5 Never
4 One time or not at all
3 Two or three times
2 Four to seven times
1 More than seven times

9. Do you eat a lot of sweets?

5 No, and I never have
4 Not often
3 Sometimes
2 I enjoy sweets and eat them often
1 I have cravings for them and have been known to "pig out"

10. Do you use antacid medications?
  5 Hardly ever
  4 Sometimes
  2 Fairly often
  1 Every day

11. Do you have dizzy spells?
  5 Never
  4 Hardly ever
  3 Sometimes
  1 Often or severe

TOTAL MINERAL IQ: ——— (transfer to page 305)

ZINC—THE SUPER MINERAL

If I had to pick the one "most vital" immune mineral, it would be zinc. Study after study has shown that zinc rebuilds every area of our immune health. Dr. Carl Pfeiffer, a researcher at the Princeton Brain Bio Center, was the first to shed light on the amazing immune-positive effects of zinc, several years ago. Unfortunately, his work was largely unrecognized until recently, when scores of studies have confirmed his work.

Dr. R. K. Chandra, an internationally acclaimed immunologist now working at MIT, treated a group of children suffering from a rare and deadly skin disease. All of the children had very poor immune responses, and they had very low levels of zinc in their blood. Remarkably, their immune responses returned to normal only a short time after these children began taking zinc supplement.

I recently treated a patient for whom zinc spelled the difference between tragedy and hope. A sixteen-year-old named Jonathan was left severely brain damaged after a tragic auto accident. This once-bright young man was paralyzed, unable to talk or communicate, dependent on intravenous nutrition. He also developed raw, ugly sores on his arms, legs, and face. My tests showed two interesting facts: first, his immune system was severely weakened and couldn't mount even an average immune response. Second, he had an abnormally low zinc level.

I started giving him zinc supplements, and an amazing change occurred. Within three weeks, his immune response was back to normal, and the angry skin sores were well on the way to healing. He began to be able to eat solid foods. After three months, his weight had increased to normal, he had learned to use a wheelchair, was more alert and, for the first time since the accident, he could communicate with others.

While zinc supplementation produces dramatic results in sick people, it also powerfully benefits those of us who seem absolutely healthy. For example:

- Zinc keeps crucial immune organs like the thymus and lymph nodes healthy
- Zinc boosts the number of your fighting T cells
- Zinc makes your T cells fight microorganisms more effectively
- Zinc strengthens your macrophages (sacvenger cells)

It is vital to get enough zinc daily because your body is able to store very little of this essential immune mineral. You do have reserves of several kinds of "strategic minerals" (calcium, iodine, and iron, for example), but scientists have discovered that the body has very small zinc reserves. Because of this, if we do not get enough zinc in our diet, or if factors in our lives deplete our small reserves, we may find ourselves with a deficiency of this immune power mineral.

ARE YOU IN A ZINC DANGER GROUP?

- Do you take oral contraceptives? If so, that may mean zinc problems, according to some research. Belgian scientists found that many women taking oral contraceptives have weak immune responses. After taking zinc for a month, the immune response of these women was completely re-energized.

- Are you pregnant? If so, research by Dr. Lucille Hurley, at the University of California, may be important for you. She found that when female animals had chronic zinc deficiencies, their offspring had severe immune system problems throughout their whole lives. Moreover, even if those offspring were given enough zinc in their diet, *their* babies still showed severe immune damage. In fact, it took *three full generations* until animals with normal immune systems could be produced. This research is so new that we don't yet know if the same thing happens in humans, but it does suggest that zinc levels are crucially important for pregnant women. If that's you or someone you love, it may be time to sound the zinc alarm.

- Are you overweight? If so, your extra fat is probably depleting your body's zinc bank accounts, throwing you into a vicious immune-fat cycle. Low zinc levels disturb your immune system, which makes you binge when eating even more. Binging further damages

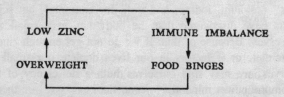

LOW ZINC → IMMUNE IMBALANCE

↑ ↓

OVERWEIGHT ← FOOD BINGES

your immune system, so that you gain weight and fall even further into the low-zinc danger zone.

Kelly's case was one of my best zinc success stories. She was one of those patients with nothing and everything wrong with her. "I feel silly coming to see you, Dr. Berger," she said. "There's really nothing specifically wrong."

Then she went on to describe a series of minor, fleeting, but bothersome ailments. In the six months before she came to see me, Kelly went through a series of low grade infections, a skin rash, and a prolonged case of athlete's foot. She suffered from recurring vaginal and urinary tract infections, and scratches she had gotten while hiking during the summer hadn't healed several weeks later. Lately, she had felt her energy flagging, and had been finding it hard to concentrate at work. Because she was an air-traffic controller, she knew she needed to be razor-sharp on the job, and she was afraid that the lack of focus she was feeling could be dangerous.

Two things stood out: first, Kelly worked in one of the most stressful of jobs. That stress meant her vitamin and mineral reserves were taxed to the limit, and zinc is especially sensitive to stress levels. Second, she was taking an oral contraceptive, further lowering her reservoir of zinc. I put her on an immune power nutrition plan that included high zinc.

Kelly called six weeks later. "I feel like a new woman! I'm back to my old self at work, and I've got more energy than I've had since I was a kid. That stuff's magic!" It's not magic, I told her, just another example of immune power healing.

There are other symptoms that low zinc can cause. If you have any of the following, you may have a zinc deficiency:

• Food doesn't taste as good as it used to
• Your sense of smell seems dull
• Your fingernails have white flecks or spots on them

- Scratches and wounds take a long time to heal
- You feel mentally dull, find it hard to concentrate
- You are losing your hair

ZINC, SEX, AND ... OYSTERS

Zinc is also a crucial factor in the male sexual system. The prostate gland and its secretions have the strongest concentrations of zinc in the body. Zinc helps to maintain potency and to make strong, healthy sperm. Oysters have earned their reputation as a potent aphrodisiac because they contain so much zinc, but wheat germ and brewer's yeast are also good sources.

These discussions about zinc don't mean that you should start taking zinc tablets indiscriminately. A recent study proved that too much zinc actually makes your immune cells less able to fight off germs. There is clearly an optimal range of zinc for peak immune health. That's why your Immune Quotient is so vital—you must find the right mineral program for your individual needs.

IRON OUT IMMUNE IMBALANCE

You've heard it said that somebody has "an iron constitution." That kind of person seems able to withstand unusual stress, eat anything, drink too much, sleep too little, be on the move constantly, and yet always manage to have vitality and energy to spare. These people are more resistant to germs, and seldom catch the colds and flu that hit the rest of us. Even if they do get sick, these lucky "iron constitution" people never get very sick; they seem to bounce back with remarkable resiliency.

There is actually a deep biological truth in the notion of an "iron constitution," because iron is one of the prime minerals you need for a super-tuned immune system. Iron enhances immunity in several ways:

- Boosts your overall resistance
- Keeps your immune tissues healthy
- Energizes your T cells
- Is a constituent of chemicals that your T cells need to kill invaders
- Makes your savenger cells pounce even more enthusiastically on bacteria

Iron has another special benefit, unlike those of the other immune nutrients which rebuild and renew only your primary immune health-keepers, the *white* blood cells. Iron also vitalizes your *red* blood cells, the back-up troops in the battle to keep you healthy and strong. The job of the red blood cells is to transport vital oxygen to all of your body's tissues, and this is necessary to life itself.

QUICK IRON CHECK

How do you know if you don't have enough iron? Look for any of these signs:

- Chronic fatigue
- Chronic malaise
- Frequent sickness or infections

JUST FOR WOMEN

You probably know that if you are menstruating, pregnant, or nursing, you require extra iron. Studies show that women need much more iron than men do, and often get only 60 percent of the iron they need. If you are also overweight, you are even more likely to have low iron.

With iron, as with most immune nutrients, you can get too much of a good thing. Dangerous bacteria need iron as much as you do, and too much iron in the blood encourages their growth. An excess of iron in the blood has been associated with overwhelming, life-threatening bacterial infections. You must be careful not to overdose on iron, for too much can be as dangerous as too little.

COPPER: THE MYSTERY MINERAL

I call copper the mystery mineral because there has been so little research done on its effects on the immune system. However, recent studies have indicated that copper does help our immune system in two important ways.

According to scientists at MIT, copper has a direct effect on several immune organs. Two groups of animals, some with sufficient copper, the others with a copper deficiency, were exposed to an infection. Look what happened:

Animal with Normal Copper (big rat)	Animal with Low Copper (little rat)
Immune tissues grew .92 percent in infection	Immune tissues grew .22 percent
Twice as many cells reacted to infection	Half as many cells reacted
Average lifespan: 25 days	Average lifespan: 7 days

Tests reported by Dr. William Beisel, at the U.S. Army Medical Research Center, show that both too little and too much copper can make infections much more severe. In addition, there is a rare disease with the unlikely name of Menkes Kinky Hair Syndrome, among infants unable to absorb copper . These babies are very vulnerable to a number of infections, and often die of them because their immune systems are unable to protect them.

Copper affects your immune system in another way. Your thyroid gland needs just the right amount of copper in order to secret its hormones. Some of these hormones directly affect the strength and distribution of the immune cells patrolling your body. If your thyroid is sluggish because of too little copper, there can be a negative ripple effect on overall immune vitality.

WHAT'S YOUR COPPER COUNT?

While copper deficiencies are not recognized as a major problem, it is very possible that you may not be getting all the copper you need. Do you show any of these signs of low copper?

- Puffiness or swelling around the ankles and wrists
- Skin problems, including eczema
- Chronic fatigue
- Frequent infections

SELENIUM AND
YOUR IMMUNE POWER

Selenium is another immune mineral about which we know far too little. We do know that a lack of selenium seems to make the immune systems far less active, particularly the scavenger cells. We also know that proper levels of selenium work with vitamin E to give us more antibodies, the ammunition that your immune soldiers use to fight infection.

Researchers at the University of California, San Diego, have also made some intriguing discoveries about this mineral. Animals prone to various kinds of cancer were fed diets high in selenium, with the result that these experimental animals had up to 88 percent fewer cases of cancer than the control group.

MEN, SEX, AND SELENIUM

Men: are you sexually active? If so, you need to make sure you get enough selenium. Men normally need more of this mineral than women do, because semen is rich in selenium, and when this mineral is discharged from the body it must be replaced for optimum sexual function. Good natural sources of selenium include bran, wheat germ, and broccoli.

BAD MINERALS: THE "HEAVIES"

Not all minerals are good for you. Some of them—like mercury, lead, cadmium, and aluminum—actually have very toxic effects. These are the so-called "heavy metal" minerals, to which we are exposed largely through environmental pollution.

How do you know if you may be exposed to heavy metals? You can start by asking yourself a few simple questions:

- Do you live next to a major roadway or airport? German searchers recently found that people living next to roadways had dangerously high levels of lead, and more incidents of cancer.
- Do you cook in aluminum pots or use aluminum foil? Certain acidic foods can leach aluminum into food.
- Do you use ceramic bowls and dishes? Glazes used in some pottery can leach lead into certain foods.
- Do you have silver fillings in your mouth? Scientists in the Netherlands found that tooth fillings can release toxic mercury into the body. Some experts believe that 30 percent of people with serious lead poisoning get it from dental fillings.
- Do you regularly take over-the-counter antacid remedies? If so, read the label: one of the main ingredients in these preparations is aluminum, which can build up in the body.

Heavy metals cause a wide variety of diseases. Mercury overdose is thought to cause blood vessel disease by eroding the walls of our arteries. It also causes bloating, fatigue, and birth defects. Lead poisoning is responsible for mental sluggishness, low appetite, vomiting, and even retardation. Mercury, lead, and cadmium can weaken your immune system.

Cadmium also appears to affect the brain, leading to

severe memory loss and diminished mental function. Some researchers believe that excess aluminum or cadmium may be factors in the development of Alzheimer's Disease (premature senility).

MINERALS AND YOUR MEMORY

Memory problems are a well-known symptom of heavy metal poisoning. Many of us are exposed to unsafe levels of these metals, particularly mercury, which is a food contaminant. There may be many more people suffering the toxic effects of heavy metal poisoning than we now recognize. Do *you* have any of these memory problems?

- Do you regularly have trouble recalling the names of people you knew last year?
- Do you misplace things more often than you used to?
- Do you ever forget the name of a familiar household object?
- Before reading this, had you already noticed any problem with your memory?
- Has a work associate, friend or family member pointed out memory problems to you in the last month?
- Have you recently felt that you are not quite as alert as you used to be?
- Have you had in the last month two embarrassing incidents wehre you forgot something important?

If you answered ''yes'' to these questions, and ''yes'' to several of the risk factors listed earlier, it is possible that you might be suffering from a toxic accumulation of heavy metals.

WHAT CAN YOU DO ABOUT IT?

The only way to remove toxic metals from the body is with a detoxification process, which involves dosages of elements that chemically bind with the metals in the body. Once the toxic metals are bound tight to the detoxifier, they are flushed out of the body together.

This is a highly controversial therapy. It is a drastic procedure done under the care of a doctor in a clinic or hospital, using intravenous drugs. Many feel the trouble, expense, and risk of the procedure outweigh its rewards.

Because I have tended to steer away from any such aggressive treatments, I do not have enough experience with intravenous detoxification to comment on the effectiveness and safety of this therapy. However, the general principle of removing heavy metal toxins from the body's tissues is medically very sound. I have used a more gentle, less invasive, less drastic way of doing it, as described on page 322.

ARE YOU GETTING ENOUGH IMMUNE POWER MINERALS?

The answer to that question is "probably not." Considering the way most people eat, getting enough of the particular immune minerals needed can be a real problem. Much of the food we eat has been processed within an inch of its life. It may look, and sometimes even taste, like nourishing food, but the odds are that most of the original vitamin and mineral content has been lost along the path of heating, cooking, drying, preserving, steaming, canning, shipping, or storing.

Most of us are in vitamin and mineral debt to our bodies. In some cases, it resembles the national debt—a perfect set-up for immune bankruptcy. What is needed is an infusion of "capital," in the form of immune power nutrients, to put your immune accounts back in the black.

MINERAL TEAMWORK AND YOUR HEALTH

In this chapter, I have discussed each of the separate minerals you need to keep your immune system healthy and fit, but I don't want to leave you with the idea that you have totally separate accounts for each vital mineral—one for iron, one for zinc, and so on. It's much more complex than that. Each immune builder works with many others, chemically combining, enhancing, and balancing, because they must all work together to produce immune power.

MINERAL SHOPPERS' TIP

When you buy mineral supplements, make sure and ask for *chelated* minerals. Chelated minerals are treated to make them much more available to your body. Non-chelated minerals may contain only one-half of the dose in a form that your body can use. Buying chelated minerals makes your health dollar go twice as far.

CHAPTER THIRTEEN

Amino Acids: The Double "A" Immune Builders

IF YOU ARE using the Immune Power Diet to lose weight, pay special attention to this chapter. There is no more exciting area of research than the dazzling discoveries now being made about how amino acids can help lower your weight *while* they boost your health.

I am going to show you how you can use some of those breakthroughs in your life. You will see:

- How an amino acid appetite suppressant can help you *directly* reduce your appetite naturally and safely
- How amino acids *indirectly* lower your appetite by eliminating destructive mood swings and food binges
- How amino acids can help you sleep better
- How you can use amino acids to relieve pain
- How amino acids help keep your memory keen and your mind alert

First, you must check your amino acid IQ.

THE AMINO ACID IQ QUIZ

1. In the last year, how often did you eat to excess?
   5 Never
   4 Once or twice
   3 3 to 5 times
   2 At least once a month
   1 Weekly or more often

2. **How is your memory?**
   5 It has always been excellent
   4 I'm occasionally absent-minded
   3 I seem to forget things more than ever, and it's annoying
   2 I definitely feel that my memory is slipping

3. **How many times in the last month have you had trouble falling asleep?**
   5 Not at all
   4 Once
   3 Four or five times
   2 Several times a week
   1 More often than that

4. **Do you have outbreaks of cold sores, shingles, or herpes?**
   5 No
   4 Sometimes I get cold sores around my mouth
   3 I have occasional outbreaks of genital herpes
   2 I often have outbreaks of genital herpes and sores on my body

5. **Do you have chronic aches and pains?**
   5 No, never
   4 I have in the past, but not lately
   3 Occasionally, but they are not serious
   2 I frequently am bothered by pain
   1 I have chronic pain that often stops me from doing things

6. **Do you have trouble controlling your weight?**
   5 No, I have always weighed the right amount
   4 I'm not overweight, but I'm always dieting
   3 My weight tends to fluctuate
   2 I gain weight very easily
   1 No matter what I've tried, I can't lose weight

7. **Do you have arthritis?**
   5 No, never
   4 Occasional or mild twinges
   3 I have moderate pain, frequently
   2 I have severe, chronic pain

8. **How well preserved are you?**
   5 I have always looked younger than my age
   4 I look good for my age
   3 I look about average for my age
   2 I'm showing my age
   1 I look older than I should

9. **How fast does your hair grow?**
   5 Very fast
   4 Moderately quickly
   3 Not as fast as it used to

10. **Do you suffer from mood and energy swings?**
    5 No, never
    4 I have in the past, but not now
    3 Yes

11. **How alert and attentive are you?**
    5 Very alert with good mental energy and organization
    4 Usually alert
    3 I catch my mind wandering often
    2 I can't think as clearly as I used to
    1 I can't seem to concentrate well any more

12. **Does your job throw your body clock off balance?**
    5 No, I work days and have regular days off each
      week
    4 Occasionally I work overtime or rotate shifts
    3 I travel often and suffer from jet lag
    2 My work schedule prevents me from sleeping
      regularly

AMINO ACIDS:
THE HELP BEHIND THE HYPE

"Amino acids" are a buzz-word today. We buy amino acid shampoos and hair conditioners, amino acid skin lotions, even amino acid cosmetics. Unfortunately, most of this is pure sales hype; few people really understand how these amino acids affect our health and weight.

In the first place, they aren't even what you think of as acids. They don't sting or eat into your skin, and they're not corrosive. You can swallow them without burning your throat. Their name comes from the fact that they belong to the chemical family of acids.

Amino acids are the building blocks of your body. You get them from the protein you eat, which is made up of combinations of different amino acids. Your body breaks protein down into its amino acid building blocks, then uses those blocks in various combinations to make your hair, fingernails, muscles, cells, tissues, and chemicals. In all, there are twenty-two different amino acids your body needs.

When I was explaining this to one of my patients, a sculptor and artist, her face lit up. "I get it, it's simple. They're just like the color chips of a mosaic. Each color is different, with its own identity and characteristics, but they all fit together to make the whole thing work!" I had to admit, after years of reading learned papers on the subject, that's still the best explanation I've ever heard.

MEET YOUR AMINO ACIDS

There are two kinds of amino acids: "non-essential," those which your body can make, and "essential" amino acids that can't be synthesized by the body. You must get the essential amino acids from what you eat, or your body won't have what it needs to do all its complex chemical tasks. Here's the round-up of all the amino acids:

Essential	Non-Essential
Histidine	Alanine
Isoleucine	Arginine
Leucine	Asparagine
Lysine	Aspartate
Methionine	Cysteine
Ornithine	Cystine
Phenylalanine	Glutamine
Threonine	Glutamate
Tryptophan	Glycine
Valine	Proline
	Serine
	Tyrosine

Scientists have known about amino acids for a long time. The news now coming from research centers across the country concerns the astounding way amino acids work to keep your immune system, and your waistline, in perfect trim. Amino acids can do four things for you: directly reduce your appetite, indirectly reduce your appetite by controlling your brain's food-mood cycle, stabilize your energy swings, and rebuild your immune fighting cells.

AMINO ACIDS AND YOUR MOOD

Amino acids help control your brain's chemical messengers, called *neurotransmitters*.

Neurotransmitters are vital for the wide range of actions, drives, and emotions that make us human. They affect hunger, thirst, sex drive, aggression, depression, sleep, anger, energy, thought, even sociability and loneliness. Neurotransmitter imbalances may create mental illnesses such as schizophrenia and several forms of depression. They also affect our higher mental processes: learning, memory, overall alertness and mental acuity. They are the chemical roots of the entire spectrum of our thoughts, actions, and feelings.

What does this have to do with what you eat? Each neurotransmitter is made up of a particular balance of amino acids. The right amino acid balance can help you avoid the depression and anxiety that often cause people to overeat and thus, indirectly, control your weight.

While I was at Harvard, much work was being done on the relationship of brain chemicals to what we eat. A Harvard research team, headed by Dr. Alan Gelenberg, found that the balance of brain chemicals depends directly on the amount and type of amino acids in our diet. In fact, they found measurable changes in brain chemistry linked to what had been eaten at the most recent meal! From this study and others, it appears that amino acids can have a profound effect on depression, anxiety, and a host of other emotions.

Because different foods contain different quantities of amino acids, it follows that what you eat exerts a strong effect on your mental state. This is what I call the ''food-mood'' connection.

AMINO ACIDS AND FOOD ABUSE

Amino acids can also help reduce the negative emotions that are at the root of food abuse. You don't have to be a psychiatrist to know what a key role mood and emotions play in destructive eating patterns. When we feel lonely, apprehensive, glum, bored, anxious, out of control, or low on self-esteem, we often look for relief at the end of a fork. This can lead to binge eating or other self-destructive, food-centered behavior—true "food abuse."

Amino acids can help! They are more gentle and much safer than powerful mind-altering drugs (the mood elevators and antidepressants) that many psychiatrists use. Those medications only mask the problem, and introduce potent chemicals into an already imbalanced brain.

By far the best and safest way to improve your mood is to do what Nature does: use amino acids to reduce negative brain chemicals and increase positive ones. Amino acids are an elegant and natural way to piggyback on Nature's flawless pharmacology, and break the food abuse cycle.

FOOD-MOOD BREAKTHROUGHS

The amino acid *tyrosine* plays a vital role in your mood. It creates a key brain messenger, *dopamine*, that controls a whole range of brain functions: thinking, memory, learning, and emotional balance. It also plays a key role in our sex drive. Furthermore, some biochemists and psychiatrists suggest that a dopamine imbalance is what causes the wild mental and emotional swings of schizophrenics. Clearly, dopamine may have a role in the ups and downs of the food abuser.

The amino acid *phenylalanine* is crucial for our body to create adrenaline, best known as the chemical that controls our fight-or-flight response. But adrenaline also does a host of other things in the body, including helping to open up the banks where you store fat. In addition, many researchers believe that people suffering from manic depression may have an adrenaline imbalance. Researchers are now finding that phenylalanine can help manic depressives. They have also had great success using this amino acid to treat other kinds of depression.

Phenylalanine is an important ingredient in the Diet Cocktail (page 321), the Jet Lag Cure (page 320), and the Brain Booster (page 320). However, this amino acid can be a problem for some people. If you have high blood pressure, or if you have the amino acid imbalance called phenylketonuria, *do not take* any formula containing phenylalanine without consulting your doctor.

Tryptophan, an essential amino acid, has been used to help people who are immobilized by certain kinds of chronic depressions. They often lack serotonin, a vital brain messenger, and tryptophan increases serotonin in the brain.

Tryptophan has another wonderful effect: it is a natural sleeping aid. Sleep is a biological essential. It rebuilds and renews the body, dissipating the toxins that accumulate after a long day of stress. However, often when you're highly stressed you may be least able to sleep, depriving your body of rest and repair just when it needs it most.

Tryptophan can help. Taken at night before bed, it is a very good way to encourage a safe, restful night's sleep. Amazingly, it won't make you sleepy if you take it during the day, but at night the body's neurochemical cycle converts tyrptophan to the brain chemicals you need to sleep well.

The amino acid *glutamine* seems to improve concentration and memory by boosting certain brain chemicals, according to Dr. Michael Lesser. Other psychiatrists have used it to help people addicted to tobacco, alcohol, or drugs because it eases anxiety during the withdrawal period. Other amino acids have been shown to lower the excess brain activity which produces epileptic-type seizures, and to potentiate certain anti-depression drugs.

Don is a perfect example of the benefits of amino acid supplementation. He was forty-two, a successful insurance agent, and the father of three children when he consulted me. He had suffered severe bouts of depression, and for the last three years, had been treated with a standard antidepressant drug. The drug had worked fairly well but not completely, and he still had some episodes of depression.

After three years, he became worried that he was becoming far too dependent on his medication, a common danger with such drugs. The more he thought about it, the more anxious and depressed he got. Wisely, he saw that he was heading into a downward spiral, so he came to my office.

Don's tests showed a lopsided amino acid balance, low in tryptophan and high in tyrosine. I prescribed a regimen to bring his amino acids back into balance. When he came back three months later, not only was his amino acid count back to normal, but he had completely stopped his antidepressant medication—for the first time in three years!

AMINO ACIDS: YOUR ENERGY THERMOSTAT

Amino acids make your body's energy thermostat—the way you absorb, digest and use protein, carbohydrates, fats, and sugars—run more smoothly. Ideally, our body should work to keep us on a smooth course of constant high energy and cheery moods. But for many people, it doesn't work that way because imbalances in the body's energy regulators cause periodic bouts of low blood sugar.

In my opinion, this is one of the most common undiagnosed medical problems in this country. The medical term for it is *reactive hypoglycemia*. This means that instead of smoothly maintaining the constant sugar and protein balance we need, the body responds jerkily, flooding itself with sugar energy ("*hyper*glycemia," or "high-sugar") then abruptly slamming on the energy brakes ("*hypo-glycemia*," or "low sugar"). We all know people who are "touchy," apt to fly off the handle, with what psychiatrists call "mood liability." Often, such people are stuck on this "hyper-hypo" seesaw, victims of a faulty energy thermostat.

People suffering reactive hypoglycemia may also be susceptible to every passing germ that comes along, and often plagued with hay fever, skin rashes, or allergies. In short, their erratic energy thermostat seems to go along with a weakened immune system. I am indebted to Dr. Jeff Bland, a noted nutritional researcher, for first bringing this constellation of symptoms to my attention.

DO YOU HAVE LOW BLOOD SUGAR?

Low blood sugar, *hypoglycemia*, is a widespread, but often overlooked, condition. Ask yourself these questions:

- Do you often suffer from "the blues," small depressions that pass quickly?
- Do you often find it difficult to concentrate before lunch or in the late afternoon?
- Does your energy go from very high to very low during the course of a normal day?
- Do you frequently get bouts of anxiety or nausea?
- At certain times in the day do you get irritable and tense for no clear reason?
- If you haven't eaten for a while, do you get severe headaches, or feel light-headed or faint?
- Are you constantly hungry?
- Are you excessively nervous or do you have trouble sleeping?
- Do you often have cold, clammy skin?

If you answered yes to three or more of these questions, you may have hidden hypoglycemia, and should ask your doctor for a five-hour glucose tolerance test.

If you recognize yourself here, the Immune Power Diet will bring you tremendous, prompt relief. Its balanced amino acid program is specifically designed to level out these exaggerated swings.

AMINO ACID TIPS

There are two key rules to help your amino acid supplements do the most good:
- Take all amino acid supplements with plenty of fluid.
- Don't take them directly before or after a heavy meal; the protein you eat will block the absorption of amino acids. Amino acids should always be taken on an empty stomach one hour before meals or at bedtime.

"DOUBLE A" CELL BUILDERS

We've seen how amino acids can smooth out your moods and regulate your energy thermostat. Now, I want to look very briefly at yet another way these amazing building blocks affect immune power.

Amino acids directly strengthen your immune fighters. This research is so new, at the very edge of the scientific frontier, that most studies have only been done on animals. Still, those studies show over and over that a strong amino acid balance increases antibodies, strengthens immune tissues, and helps the body fight infection.

A very promising amino acid for immune power is *arginine*. Preliminary studies indicate that it stimulates the immune tissues, and on-going research is seeking to define arginine's role as a potential amino acid immune booster.

We are now on the brink of understanding how and why amino acids improve our immunity. The complete story of amino acids and the immune system simply can't be written yet—it is a story only time will finish.

NEWSFLASH—AMINO ACIDS AND PAIN

As this book is going to press, brand new research from England shows that an amino acid, *d-phenylalanine*, provides significant pain relief for patients with a variety of chronic pain conditions, including lower back pain, herpes, and post-surgical discomfort. (This is a different amino acid than the form of phenylalanine I discussed earlier.)

TEAMWORK IS CRUCIAL FOR THE "DOUBLE A" TEAM

Teamwork is the secret of using amino acids to boost your immune power. More than any other immune power nutrient, these substances must be perfectly balanced. In fact, many amino acids, like lysine and arginine, are meant to work in precisely paired ratios. To be effective as brain messengers, energy thermostat regulators and immune boosters, amino acids must be in a balanced equilibrium.

However, these powerful immune enhancers can also create powerful problems if you take them carelessly. Improper self-dosing is bad medicine, a one-way road to real immune trouble.

Disrupting amino acid balance is the chemical equivalent of dropping putty into the works of a fine Swiss watch—with even more serious results.

This is the reason that all of the recipes, as well as the entire Immune Power Diet, use safe, complementary, balanced amino acids. For the few conditions where I prescribe separate amino acids, they are *safe in the doses I have given.*

Some people have problems absorbing or making certain amino acids. One of the most frequent of these conditions, called *phenylketonuria*, occurs when the body is unable to break down the amino acid phenylalanine, which then builds up causing mental retardation. If you have any amino acid-related problems then any changes in your amino acids could be dangerous. Consult your physician.

It is essential—absolutely vital—that you follow exactly the recommendations I've given here. *Taking these chemicals willy nilly, in any way that throws off your body's fine chemical balance, can be extremely dangerous.* Remember, every time you pick up one of these powerful chemicals, you should treat it as though it were stamped: HANDLE WITH CARE.

CHAPTER FOURTEEN

Using Your IQ (Immune Quotient)

YOU'RE ALMOST READY to figure out your Comprehensive Immune Quotient and start on your individual rebuilding program of vitamins, minerals, and amino acids.

But first, you have three short quizzes left to take. Your life-style, stress, and exercise levels must be evaluated to give you the most *specific and helpful* IQ possible.

WHAT'S YOUR IMMUNE LIFE-STYLE?

Your immune health is affected by everything about you—your genes, activities, habits, occupation, and a host of other factors.

THE LIFE-STYLE IQ QUIZ

---

1. **Is there a history of problem drinking in your family?**
   5 No
   4 One close relative
   3 More than one close relative
   2 I used to have a drinking problem
   1 I currently have a drinking problem

2. **On the average, how many cigarettes a day do you smoke?**
   5 None, and I never have
   4 None now, but I used to smoke regularly
   3 Less than half a pack
   2 About a pack a day
   1 More than a pack a day

3. **How many times in the past year have you been hospitalized?**
   5 Not at all
   4 Once, for a minor problem or childbirth
   3 More than once, but only minor problems, no surgery
   2 Once for major illness or surgery
   1 More than once for major illness or surgery

4. **Does your family have a history of cancer, or other immune-suppressive disorders?**
   5 No history
   3 One immediate family member
   2 More than one immediate family member
   1 I myself have had such disorders

5. **How many prescription medicines are you now taking?**
   5 None
   4 One or two
   3 Three or four
   2 Five or six
   1 More than six

6. **Do you use illicit drugs?**
   5 No
   4 Not now, but I used to
   3 Yes, but infrequently
   2 Yes, regularly
   1 I am/have been a problem drug user

7. **How often do you eat cured or processed meats? (i.e., bacon, sausage, luncheon meats)**
   5 Never
   4 Very infrequently
   3 At least once a week
   2 Several times a week
   1 At least once a day

8. **When you shop, do you read food labels for additives?**
   5 Yes, and I avoid foods with a lot of additives
   4 Sometimes, but I don't always bother
   2 Very rarely
   1 I don't really care at all

9. **Based on your recent health, do you expect to get sick in the next six months?**
   5 Definitely not
   4 Probably not
   3 Maybe one minor cold or flu
   2 Probably more than one minor illness
   1 I am sick right now

10. **Are you taking antibiotics for any medical problem?**
    5 No
    4 Not now, but within the last year
    3 Off and on
    1 Yes

11. **Do you have allergy problems?**
    5 Never
    4 I used to, but no longer
    3 Mild, seasonal problems only
    2 Mild year-round problems
    1 Allergies are a real problem for me

12. **How do you describe your health?**
    5 Excellent, as always
    4 Better than before, and still improving
    3 Usually good
    2 Not as good as it used to be
    1 Poor, or getting worse

13. **How regular are your bowel movements?**
    5 Very regular
    4 Usually regular
    3 Bouts with diarrhea
    2 Not very regular
    1 Often constipated

14. **Which best describes your attitudes about health?**
    5 The way I live affects my health. I make it a point to treat my body well.
    4 Though usually in good health, I'm destined to be sick occasionally.
    3 My health is about average, and there's not much I can do about it.
    2 In 20 years, I will be much less healthy than I am now.
    1 I worry a lot about my health.

15. **Overall, your diet is:**
    5 Excellent
    4 Better than average
    3 About average
    2 Could be better
    1 Poor

TOTAL LIFE-STYLE IQ SCORE ——— (transfer to page 306)

STRESS: THE HIDDEN KILLER

Stress is one of the most powerful, and most insidious, factors that can hurt your immune system. We know that there are powerful links between your mental state, stress, and your immune health. Stress depletes a whole alphabet of vitamins—A, B, C, D, and E—as well as minerals such as zinc, calcium, iron, magnesium, potassium, molybdenum, and sulphur. You've seen how necessary these are for your overall health, so it comes as no surprise that high stress means less immune power. For that reason, it's crucial you assess your stress level for your overall Immune Quotient.

YOUR STRESS IQ QUIZ

1. **Overall, how satisfied are you with your career or work?**
   5 I am doing exactly what I want to do
   4 I am generally happy, but sometimes dissatisfied
   3 I don't find much satisfaction in my work
   2 I am not at all satisfied, but I am trying to change that
   1 I feel trapped in what I do

2. **What big changes have you made in your life in the last year?**
   5 Nothing too serious
   4 Changed jobs/school; got married/engaged; moved in with lover
   3 Got divorced/separated/broke up with lover; major career change; moved to a new area
   2 A close relative or friend died
   1 Spouse or lover died

3. **When did you last do something just for fun?**
   5 Today
   4 Within the last few days
   3 Within the last month
   2 I don't remember
   1 Fun is just for children; I don't have the time

4. **How stressful is your job or daily routine?**
   5 Enough to be challenging, which I enjoy
   4 Pretty stressful, but I'm usually able to control it
   3 Sometimes gets too high pressure
   2 Very stressful, and I'm starting to feel the effects
   1 Too stressful; I really need a break

5. **Do you have ulcers or stomach problems?**
   5 No, never
   4 Not now, but I have at times
   3 I think I may, but I haven't been checked yet
   2 Yes, occasionally
   1 Yes, they are a chronic problem

6. **How often do you express your inner feelings with words?**
   5 Always—I need to
   4 Usually
   3 Sometimes, but it's hard
   2 Only when there's no choice
   1 Never—it's just not my style

7. **How do you normally react to a high-stress situation?**
   5 Use mental techniques or relaxation to calm down
   4 Try to tell myself to calm down, but can't always
   3 "Explode," then feel better
   2 Take it out on someone else, but feel bad later
   1 Keep it to myself

8. **Right now: Are you satisfied with your life?**
   5 Yes, very satisfied overall
   4 Pretty satisfied, but there are some problems
   3 Not always satisfied, but try to take things one day
     at a time
   2 Things aren't very good, but are getting better
   1 I wish I were a different person

9. **Do you have a close friend or family member to confide in?**
   5 Yes, definitely, more than one
   4 Probably one for sure
   3 Not sure
   2 Probably not
   1 Definitely not

10. **Do you think of yourself as "in love" right now?**
    5 Yes, and I'm ecstatic
    4 Yes, in a quiet way
    3 Not right now, but I have been
    2 Not yet, but I hope I will be
    1 No, and I wonder if I ever will be

11. **Which is your energy level?**
    5 More than enough energy
    4 Enough energy, but not any extra
    3 I tire after physical or mental activity
    2 I don't have as much energy as I used to
    1 I'm often or always fatigued

12. **How much sleep do you get?**
    5 Six to eight hours, and I always feel rested
    4 Sometimes less, but I usually catch up
    3 Less than I'd like, and I sometimes feel like I need
      a nap
    2 Not as much sleep as I think I need
    1 I sleep poorly, I am almost always tired

13. How often do you have headaches?
  5 At most, one or two mild ones a year
  4 Less than one a month, and always mild
  3 Occasional headaches, mild to severe
  2 Frequent headaches
  1 Headaches are a real problem for me

14. Has anyone in your immediate family had heart problems?
  5 No
  4 Only one family member
  3 More than one immediate family member
  2 I have high blood pressure
  1 I have had angina or a heart attack

TOTAL STRESS IQ SCORE ———— (transfer to page 306)

EXERCISE AND IMMUNE FITNESS

The amount of exercise you get can also affect your immune health. The following quiz has been designed in conjunction with the sports medicine experts at the Biofitness Institute, New York's most acclaimed sports medicine group, to help you assess your own exercise IQ.

YOUR EXERCISE IQ QUIZ

1. How often do you exercise vigorously for at least 15 to 20 minutes?
  5 More than four times a week
  4 About three times a week
  3 Once or twice a week
  2 Not regularly
  1 I don't exercise

2. **Which is the best description of your blood pressure?**
   5 It is low
   4 It is normal
   3 It used to be high, but is now normal
   2 It is too high occasionally
   1 It is consistently too high

3. **What is your pulse rate after 15 minutes of rest?**
   5 Below 65
   4 65 to 70
   3 71 to 75
   2 76 to 85
   1 Above 85

4. **Do you engage in outdoor activities?**
   5 Yes, as much as possible
   4 Often
   3 Sometimes
   2 Not really, only rarely
   1 Never

5. **How do you feel after strenuous exercise?**
   5 Great
   4 Good, sometimes a little tired
   3 I always need to rest for a while
   2 Fatigued, exhausted
   1 Ill, nauseated

6. **How warm are you in really cold weather?**
   5 Fine, cold is not a problem for me
   4 Usually not a problem
   3 I get occasional chills, but nothing severe
   2 I get cold very easily
   1 I can't keep warm when it's cold, no matter what

7. **When was the last time you walked two miles without stopping?**
   5 More than once within the past week
   4 Once within the past week
   3 Within the past month
   2 Within the past three months
   1 I don't remember

8. **How is your physique today compared to five years ago?**
   5 The same, I have always been in good shape
   4 I am in better shape today than I was five years ago
   3 I am a little more out of shape than I was five years ago
   2 I am considerably more out of shape than five years ago
   1 I have never been in good shape

TOTAL EXERCISE IQ SCORE ——— (transfer to page 306)

YOUR COMPREHENSIVE IQ CHART

CALCULATE YOUR OWN IQ

Write your scores for the IQ quizzes here:

IQ CHART

		If your	You are in
Vitamin IQ	———		
Mineral IQ	———	Total IQ is:	IQ category:
Amino Acid IQ	———	351–390	A

Life-style IQ	———	276–350	B
Stress IQ	———	196–275	C
Exercise IQ	———	121–195	D
Total IQ	———	78–120	E

If You Have an "A" Level IQ:

If you are in the "A" category, CONGRATULATIONS! You are probably in the best immune shape possible. For you, the optimal doses you need to stay in top immune condition are listed on page 308. You can add to these any other specific Immune Boosters (page 314) necessary for your life-style.

If You Have a "B" Level IQ:

Good news! Your IQ test shows that you are already in strong immune shape, but you still can put yoruself in even better immune tune. You will get best results by following the program on page 309. Take this program for six weeks, then you will graduate to the "A" program, on page 308. This is your ongoing maintenance dose, with which you can stay as long as you like. When you are at A level, you can add any specific Immune Boosters you wish.

If You Have a "C" Level IQ:

If you are in the "C" category, you are in the ideal group to benefit from Immune Power nutrients. To get the best and safest results, you have to build up your supplements in a four step program. For the next five days, follow the "A" program on page 308. Then, for the five days following that, follow the "B" program on page 309. Now you are ready to re-energize your immune system: Stay on the "C" program on page 310 for the next four weeks.

Then, reverse the process. For four more weeks, follow the "B" program. Finally, maintain with the "A" program. You can stay on this as long as you like and at this point you can add any specific Immune Boosters.

If You Have a "D" Level IQ:

You can expect to see real, positive changes with the Immune Power Program. But you cannot begin the high "D" doses suddenly. You need to build your body up to get the best and safest results from the program. Start first with five days of the "A" program on page 308. Then for five days on the "B" program on page 309 followed by five days on the "C" program on page 310. You are now ready to rebuild. Stay on the "D" program on page 311 for four weeks. Then go four weeks on the "B" program. Finally, reduce to the "A" program, where you can stay as long as you like, maintaining your new immune health at your optimal dose level. You can now add any specific Immune Boosters as needed.

If You Have an "E" Level IQ:

Of all the groups, you have the most to gain from the Immune Power program! However, DO NOT begin suddenly at the "E" level doses. Instead, build up gradually to get your body used to it. Start first with five days of the "A" program on page 308. Then for five days each, follow the "B" program (page 309), the "C" program (page 310), and the "D" program (Page 311). Now you are ready for serious immune building. Stay on the "E" program for four weeks. Then, reduce your supplements to "C" program levels for four weeks. Follow this with four weeks on the "B" program. Now you are ready for the "A" program, which you continue as long as you like— you are maintaining your immune power at your optimal dose level. Only at this point may you add any specific Immune Boosters.

YOUR IQ-BASED NUTRIENT PROGRAM

Now that you have found your Immune Quotient, turn to nutrient programs especially tailored to each IQ category. Remember to follow exactly the specific doses in each IQ category.

"A" LEVEL IQ

Vitamins:

Vitamin A	10,000 IU
B₁ Thiamine	100 mg.
B₂ Riboflavin	100 mg.
B₃ Niacin	100 mg.
B₅ Pantothenic Acid	200 mg.
B₆ Pyridoxine	50 mg.
PABA	250 mg.
B₁₂	200 mcg.
Folic Acid	400 mcg.
Choline	200 mg.
Inositol	200 mg.
Biotin	100 mcg.
Vitamin C	2,000 mg.
Vitamin D	400 IU
Vitamin E	400 IU
Bioflavonoids:	
Rutin	400 mg.
Hesperidin Complex	400 mg.

Minerals:

Calcium	400 mg.
Magnesium	200 mg.
Iron	10 mg.
Zinc	50 mg.
1-Selenomethionine	100 mcg.

Amino Acids:

N, N-Dimethylglycine Hydrochloride   100 mg.

Add any extra Immune Life-style Booster doses here from page 314:

————
————
————
————
————
————

mg. = milligram
mcg. = microgram

"B" LEVEL IQ

Vitamins:

Vitamin A	15,000 IU
B$_1$ Thiamine	200 mg.
B$_2$ Riboflavin	150 mg.
B$_3$ Niacin	100 mg.
B$_5$ Pantothenic Acid	250 mg.
B$_6$ Pyridoxine	75 mg.
PABA	300 mg.
B$_{12}$	250 mcg.
Folic Acid	400 mcg.
Choline	250 mg.
Inositol	250 mg.
Biotin	200 mcg.
Vitamin C	3,000 mg.
Vitamin D	400 IU
Vitamin E	400 IU
Bioflavonoids:	
Rutin	400 mg.
Hesperidin Complex	400 mg.

Minerals:

Calcium	600 mg.
Magnesium	300 mg.
Iron	15 mg.
Zinc	50 mg.
1-Selenomethionine	150 mcg.

Amino Acids:

N, N-Dimethylglycine Hydrochloride	100 mg.
L-Cysteine	1,000 mg.
(take with C)	

mg. = milligram
mcg. = microgram

"C" LEVEL IQ

Vitamins:

Vitamin A	15,000 IU
B$_1$ Thiamine	250 mg.
B$_2$ Riboflavin	150 mg.
B$_3$ Niacin	200 mg.
B$_5$ Pantothenic Acid	300 mg.
B$_6$ Pyridoxine	100 mg.
PABA	500 mg.
B$_{12}$	300 mcg.
Folic Acid	500 mcg.
Choline	300 mg.
Inositol	300 mg.
Biotin	300 mcg.
Vitamin C	4,000 mg.
Vitamin D	600 IU
Vitamin E	600 IU
Bioflavonoids:	
Rutin	500 mg.
Hesperidin Complex	500 mg.

Minerals:

Calcium	800 mg.
Magnesium	400 mg*
Manganese	5 mg.
Iron	20 mg.
Zinc	75 mg.
1-Selenomethionine	200 mcg.
Copper	0.1 mg.

Amino Acids:

N, N-Dimethylglycine Hydrochloride	200 mg.
L-Arginine (bedtime)	1,000 mg.
L-Orinthine	1,000 mg.
L-Cysteine	1,000 mg.
(take with C)	

mg. = milligram
mcg. = microgram

* If you have a kidney malfunction, reduce this to 300 mg.

"D" LEVEL IQ

Vitamins:

Vitamin A	20,000 IU
B₁ Thiamine	300 mg.
B₂ Riboflavin	200 mg.
B₃ Niacin	300 mg.
B₅ Pantothenic Acid	500 mg.
B₆ Pyridoxine	150 mg.
PABA	750 mg.
B₁₂	400 mcg.
Folic Acid	600 mcg.
Choline	400 mg.
Inositol	400 mg.
Biotin	400 mcg.

Vitamin C	5,000 mg.
Vitamin D	600 IU
Vitamin E	800 IU
Bioflavonoids:	
Rutin	500 mg.
Hesperidin Complex	500 mg.

Minerals:

Calcium	1,000 mg.
Magnesium	500 mg.*
Manganese	10 mg.
Iron	25 mg.
Zinc	75 mg.
1-Selenomethionine	250 mcg.
Copper	0.1 mg.
Chromium	100 mcg.
Phosphorous	150 mg.
Potassium	99 mg.

Amino Acids:

N, N-Dimethylglycine	
Hydrochloride	200 mg.
L-Arginine (bedtime)	2,000 mg.
L-Ornithine	1,000 mg.
L-Cysteine	1,500 mg.
(take with C)	

mg. = milligram
mcg. = microgram

* If you have a kidney malfunction, reduce this to 300 mg.

"E" LEVEL IQ

Vitamins:

Vitamin A	20,000 IU
B₁ Thiamine	500 mg.
B₂ Riboflavin	250 mg.
B₃ Niacin	400 mg.
B₅ Pantothenic Acid	750 mg.
B₆ Pyridoxine	200 mg.
PABA	1,000 mg.
B₁₂	500 mcg.
Folic Acid	800 mcg.
Choline	500 mg.
Inositol	500 mg.
Biotin	500 mcg.
Vitamin C	6,000 mg.
Vitamin D	1,000 IU
Vitamin E	1,000 IU
Bioflavonoids:	
Rutin	
Hesperidin	

Minerals:

Calcium	1,200 mg.
Magnesium	600 mg.*
Manganese	20 mg.
Iron	25 mg.
Zinc	100 mg.
1-Selenomethionine	300 mcg.
Copper	0.2 mg.
Chromium	200 mcg.
Phosphorous	200 mg.
Potassium	99 mg.

Amino Acids:

N, N-Dimethylglycine	
Hydrochloride	300 mg.

L-Arginine (bedtime)	3,000 mg.
L-Orinthine	2,000 mg.
L-Cysteine	2,000 mg.
(take with C)	

mg. = milligram
mcg. = microgram

* If you have a kidney malfunction, reduce this to 300 mg.

IMMUNE LIFE-STYLE BOOSTERS

Each of us has specific factors in our lives that mean we need more of specific nutrients—above and beyond the regular IQ doses. If you fall into any of the categories below, add these extra boosters to your *final* IQ maintenance dose—the "A" level doses.

But remember: Add Life-style Boosters ONLY when you are maintaining in the "A" category. They are meant to work with your ongoing maintenance dose. Do not add them to the rebuilding doses in the "B," "C," "D," or "E" categories.

FOR MEN

1-Selenomethionine	50 mcg.
Zinc	30 mg.
Vitamin E	200 IU

FOR WOMEN

Folic Acid	200 mcg.
Calcium	500 mg.
Magnesium	500 mg.
Iron	10 mg.

If you take oral contraceptives:

Vitamin B_6	25 mg.
Vitamin C	500 mg.
Folic Acid	400 mcg.
Zinc	25 mg.
Vitamin E	100 IU
Chromium	25 mcg.

If you are taking a course of antibiotics:

Folic Acid	100 mcg.
Vitamin B_{12}	20 mcg.
Vitamin C	500 mg.

If you are taking diuretics or high blood pressure medication:

Magnesium	100 mg.
Zinc	20 mg.

If you exercise heavily (20 minutes three times a week or more):

B complex 100 (yeast free)	1 tablet per day
Magnesium	100 mg.
Vitamin E	200 IU
Vitamin C	1,000 mg
Calcium	200 mg.
Potassium	50 mg.
Iron	5 mg.

FOR YOUR OWN GOOD

So far, I've talked about what you can do on the Immune Power Diet. Now it's time to take just a moment for a few warnings.

Some people have diseases or genetic conditions which make it unadvisable for them to take certain supplements in the Immune Quotient program. Specifically, if you have any of the problems I mention here, it is vital that you *avoid* the nutrients listed below.

Of course, before you start the Immune Power program, I recommend you consult your own doctor to make sure you don't have any hidden problem that could create problems with any of the supplements listed. Do not be surprised if many of your physicians are not familiar with immune power nutritional supplementations, as much of this information is new and not in their area of expertise.

- If you are pregnant, DO NOT TAKE more than 50 milligrams of vitamin B$_6$ on a daily basis. *All pregnant women should consult their own doctor before starting on this, or any other, supplementation regimen.*
- If you *regularly take medication* or are under care for any chronic medical condition (especially heart disease, high blood pressure, or diabetes), your IQ supplements may mean you need less medication. Discuss this with your physican before taking any of the IQ supplements.
- *Adolescents* should not take these supplements without checking with their own physicians.
- If you have *heart disease*, consult your doctor to make sure how much vitamin D to take.
- If you have *rheumatic heart disease*, vitamin E can worsen your condition. Consult your doctor before taking it.
- If you have a *kidney malfunction*, DO NOT TAKE more than 300 mg. of magnesium on a daily basis. Also, do not take more than 500 mg. of vitamin C.
- If you have *diabetes, stomach ulcers, glaucoma*, or *liver problems*, consult your own doctor before taking Niacin.

- If you have *high blood pressure*, DO NOT TAKE 1-Phenylalanine without informing your doctor, as it can elevate blood pressure. If you do take it, start with small doses, 100 mg. or so, then build up gradually, while checking your blood pressure frequently.

- If you are a *diabetic*, DO NOT TAKE vitamin C or B_1, or the amino acid L-Cysteine, without consulting your physician. They can interfere with insulin in the body.

- If you take a drug for *Parkinson's Disease*, DO NOT TAKE vitamin B_6 without consulting your physician. The vitamin can interfere with the action of L-Dopa type drugs in the brain, and actually make your symptoms worse.

- If you have *phenylketonuria*, DO NOT TAKE 1-Phenylalanine.

- If you have *any amino acid imbalance condition*, or problems with absorption or synthesis of amino acids, DO NOT TAKE any amino acids without consulting your physician.

- When taking the amino acid L-Cysteine, follow the recommended dosage. It must be taken in a 1:3 ratio with vitamin C.

TOO MUCH OF A GOOD THING

The supplements in the IQ programs will make you healthier as will the suggestions for specific vitamins, minerals, fatty acids or amino acids I recommend in the next chapter for specific conditions like gray hair, insominia, appetite suppression, or pre-menstrual syndrome. However, there is such a thing as too much of a good thing, and you must be careful not to overdose yourself.

You should wait until you are maintaining yourself on

the "A" level dose before you take any of the specific remedies I suggest in the last chapter. DO NOT ADD them to the rebuilding doses in the "B," "C," "D," or "E" categories. The same is true for the Immune Lifestyle Boosters. These extra doses are meant to be used ONLY when you are maintaining in the "A" category.

CHAPTER FIFTEEN

Insiders' Immune Power Tips

I'M GOING TO treat you now as if you were sitting on the other side of the desk in my office, and pass on some tips that only my patients, the Immune Power Diet insiders, get.

These special nutrient supplements have been created to help specific patients with specific problems. They have repeatedly been tested and found to be safe and effective.

But, and this is a very big BUT, do not use any of these formulas until you are in perfect immune tune—that is, on the A level supplement program. *To do so at any other level will interfere with your progress toward maximum immunity and may actually impair your system.*

For A levelers only, here are some tips on a natural *sleep aid*, an amino acid *brain booster*, a *cure for jet lag*, a natural *appetite suppressant, a heavy metal detoxification program*, and a formula for the *relief of pre-menstrual tension*. You'll also find a *"morning after" formula*, and a nutrient plan that will help your body fight off *the effect of caffeine and cigarettes*. I'm even going to tell you how to fight *prematurely graying hair!*

A SAFE, NATURAL SLEEP AID

Don't use powerful hypnotic or narcotic drugs. Try this natural amino acid recipe to help you get the rest you need.

500 mg. l-Tryptophan six hours after rising.

500 mg. l-Tryptophan (on an empty stomach) one hour before bedtime.

JET LAG CURE

Being a frequent flyer may gain you free trips on the airlines, but it wreaks havoc on your health. People who frequently fly long distances have been shown to get sick more, often with immune deficiency related problems. Scientists think this may be due to the damaging effect of constantly setting and resetting the body's biological clock.

You can use amino acids to lessen jet lag and reduce the toll that resetting your biological clock takes on your body. The next time you have a long plane flight—particularly west to east, which is hardest on your body's rhythms—try the following:

> 100 mg. vitamin B_6
> 1 gram l-Tyrosine
> 1 gram vitamin C

Take this just before bed when you have landed or, if you will be sleeping during the flight, just before you fall asleep. Try to take it on an empty stomach. If it doesn't work, or if you get a headache, substitute an equal dose of phenylalanine for the tyrosine.

AMINO ACID BRAIN BOOSTER

L-Phenylalanine has been found to improve higher mental functions, including memory, learning, motivation, and alertness. Do you have a test, or speech, or important meeting where you need to be at peak form? If so, take the following, on an empty stomach, early in the day:

> 1 gram 1-Phenylalanine
> 1 gram vitamin C
> 200 mg. vitamin B_6

THE DOUBLE "A" APPETITE SUPPRESSANT

One of the best ways you can use amino acids to control your weight is in the form of what I call my "Diet Cocktail," a special formula I have developed that uses natural vitamins and amino acids to reduce appetite. In the past, appetite suppressants have gotten a deservedly bad reputation, because they were dangerous, and prescribed additive drugs such as amphetamines. Many physicians prescribed these drugs without adequate attention to their serious side effects.

This "Diet Cocktail" avoids all of that. Using natural ingredients, it works with the body's own appetite control center in the brain. You will join hundreds of overweight patients in a toast to good health with this "cocktail." Here's the recipe

> 1000 mg. vitamin C
> 500 mg. 1-Phenylalanine
> 100 mg. vitamin B_6

For best results, take this just before bed, on an empty stomach. You will find it helps lower your appetite the next day.

Some people are sensitive to the phenylalanine in this "cocktail." If this is a problem you can substitute the same dose of the amino acid *l-Tyrosine*. Whichever way works for you, the "cocktail" will give your body a new "happy hour" to look forward to because your body will be so happy to get a safe, effective way to eat less!

HEAVY METAL DETOXIFICATION PROGRAM

This is a safe, low-level regime designed to be followed for six weeks. Developed to treat high levels of mercury, the metal you are most likely to have been exposed to, this detoxification program requires no intravenous treatment, and no hospitilization. Instead, each day take:

- 300 milligrams of 1-Glutathione (a synthetic amino acid)
- 3 grams of L-Cysteine
- 9 grams of vitamin C
- 300 micrograms of 1-Selenomethionine

The Vitamin C in this formula removes lead from the brain and bones, and helps prevent build-up of heavy minerals by keeping them in solution so your body can eliminate them. The amino acid L-Cysteine strongly binds heavy metals. (Remember that L-Cysteine and vitamin C must be taken in the recommended 1:3 ratio). Selenium is especially protective against mercury.

Not everybody ought to take this program. How do you know if you should? Two reasons: If your comprehensive IQ was originally in either the "D" or "E" group, AND if you believe that you are exposed to high levels of lead or mercury, you may want to try it.

If so, follow these two essential rules:

1) You must be at the lowest maintenance doses of supplements (A level), during the time you are on the detoxifying program. *If you follow the detoxification program without reducing your other supplements, you may suffer symptoms of vitamin, mineral, or amino acid overdose.*

2) DO NOT follow this detoxifying program without consulting your own doctor first. It is highly unlikely that a physician not specifically trained in vitamin therapy will be familiar with the detoxifying effects of these vitamins. However, it is essential to have your blood chemistry professionally monitored throughout this treatment. If your physician is not willing to do this, you should *not* try this detoxification program. Readers of this book may contact me for a list of local physicians trained in this area.

NATURAL RELIEF FOR PRE-MENSTRUAL SYNDROME

Minerals can help if you are one of the millions of women who get severe pre-menstrual symptoms. We have only recently recognized the variety those symptoms can take: anxiety, irritability, headaches, depression, a craving for sweets, weight gain, even tender breasts. If you feel any of the symptoms listed here, take the mineral and vitamin supplements listed.

1. For best results, take ten days before your period starts.
2. If you have several of these symptoms, decide which symptom is most severe, and take the supplements I recommend for that problem. *Do not take supplements from more than one symptom category.*

If you suffer from . . . Take these supplements

Anxiety/	Vitamin E	800 IU/day
Irritability	Vitamin B₁	250 mg./day
	Vitamin B₆	400 mg./day
	Magnesium	500 mg./day
Headaches, dizziness,	Vitamin E	800 IU/day
sweet cravings,	Vitamin B₁	250 mg./day
weakness	Vitamin B₆	400 mg./day
	Vitamin C	2 grams (3 × daily)
	Chromium	200 mcg./day
Painful, tender	Vitamin B₁	250 mg./day
breasts	Vitamin E	800 IU/day
	Magnesium	500 mg./day
	Evening	
	Primrose Oil	2 grams (3 × daily)
Depression, confusion,	Vitamin E	800 IU/day
fatigue, lethargy	Vitamin B₁	250 mg./day
	Vitamin B₆	400 mg./day
	Zinc	30 mg./day
	*1-Tryptophan	1000 mg./day

* If you feel no response, or get headaches, switch to the same dose of another amino acid, 1-Phenylalanine.

ARE YOU BOOZE-PROOF?

Most of us know about alcohol's more popular effects, but few are aware that it can very severely deplete our mineral and vitamin stores. As you metabolize alcohol, your body flushes a tremendous amount of water through your kidneys to eliminate alcohol from the blood, and that water also carries the water-soluble minerals with it—potassium, sodium, iron, zinc, copper. That mineral imbalance is part of what creates the awful "morning after" feeling, and explains why many drinkers are prone to anxiety, fatigue, insomnia, low energy, irritability, confusion, and depression.

You don't have to drink a lot to feel these effects—two pre-dinner cocktails can leave you feeling tired and ill the next day. Moderate drinking is not generally considered harmful *if you carefully replace those lost vitamins and minerals.*

A MORNING AFTER FORMULA

If you drink alcohol, here is a formula that can help replace the vital nutrients alcohol flushes from your system. The morning after a hard night, take:

> 100 mg. vitamin B_1 (Thiamine)
> 100 mg. vitamin B_2 (Riboflavin)
> 50 mg. vitamin B_6
> 250 mcg. vitamin B_{12}
> 1,000 mg. vitamin C
> 50 mg. Zinc

COFFEE, COLA, AND MINERALS

What do coffee, tea, chocolate, and many soft drinks have in common? They all contain caffeine, which may be sapping your body's vital minerals. In a complicated biochemical process caffeine "tricks" your kidneys and they pump out essential mineral and vitamin reserves. That loss, plus the primary central nervous system effect of caffeine creates a wide range of symptoms; "coffee nerves," poor concentration, insomnia, and a less-vigilant immune system.

A CAFFEINE ANTIDOTE

Whether you are a two-cups-before-you-open-your-eyes kind of coffee drinker, or you just drink a cola or two at work, here's a formula to help you replace the nutrients destroyed by caffeine.

> 1,000 mg. vitamin C
> 50 mg. Zinc
> 400 mg. Calcium
> 500 mg. Magnesium
> B Complex Vitamin

VITAMINS FOR SMOKERS

We've all heard lots about the harm smoking can do, but what you may not know is that smoking depletes the body's vitamin reserves. Tobacco smoke actually robs the body of vitamins like Thiamine (B_1), Pyridoxine (B_6), and C which power the immune system and also keep the nervous system ticking smoothly and efficiently.

If you're not minding your B's and C's, you get more anxious, irritable and jumpy—that's what "smoker's nerves" or "nic fits" are all about. More importantly, your immune system is denied the vitamins it needs to protect you just when you need it most—when you inhale the carcinogens associated with cigarette smoke.

Each cigarette you smoke destroys an average of 25 milligrams of vitamin C. If you are a two-pack-a-day smoker, you will lose, 1,000 mg. which is more vitamin C than most of us take in a day. That cumulative loss sets off an insidous cycle. The more you smoke, the more immune strength you need, but the less you have. The cycle gets worse, because the more stress you feel the greater your urge to smoke.

Vitamin A also has very direct benefits for smokers. A recent international study showed that smokers with a vitamin A deficiency are much more likely to develop cancers of the lung, bronchial tubes, and mouth than smokers whose vitamin A levels are normal. This mean it's crucial for smokers to eat a lot of vitamin A-rich foods such as liver, egg yolks, and a variety of green leafy and yellow vegetables.

FOR SMOKERS . . .

If you smoke, you may lack *several vitamins*. Here is a regime that I recommend for my patients who still smoke:
Each morning, take:

> 20,000 IU vitamin A
> 400 IU vitamin E
> 1,000 mg. vitamin C
> 50 mg. Zinc
> 100 mg. thiamine (B_1)
> 100 mg. riboflavin (B_2)
> 50 mg. pyridoxine (B_6)
> 250 mcg. cobalamine (B_{12})

AWAY WITH THE GRAY!

Do you remember my patient Kirk, whose hair went gray at the age of only twenty-six? What happened to Kirk may happen to you if you are not getting the proper vitamins.

But, like Kirk, you may reverse premature graying and restore your natural color without rinses or dyes.

Hair color is strongly influenced by the B vitamins, pantothenic acid, PABA, and folic acid, which are necessary to produce pigment. Taking these vitamins may give you a natural, safe, long-lasting way to get rid of the gray and regain your youthful appearance.

If you are prematurely gray, try this safe, effective formula daily for three months—and see if you don't notice a change for the better.

> 300 mg. pantothenic acid (vitamin B_5)
> 1,000 mg. PABA
> 600 mcg. folic acid

CHAPTER SIXTEEN

Conclusion: Making Immune Power a Part of Your Life

ON THE first page of this book I congratulated you on the decision you made when you picked up this book: your decision to create a healthier (and probably thinner) you. Now that you know your way towards the goal of rebuilding your immune health, I want to leave behind all the scientific studies and findings, to concentrate on something much more interesting: You.

You, after all, are the single most important part of this diet. Not the studies, not your immune cells, not even your IQ—but you as a person. To make immune power work for you, and to enjoy the sweeping improvements in health and weight loss that come with it, this program has to work in your life, the way you want to live it.

That means that nobody but *you* can make the commitment that will allow you to give yourself the health you deserve. When I say "commitment," I don't mean to me, or to this book, or to any specific program, but to a very simple idea: enjoying the rest of your life in the best possible health.

The Immune Power Diet commitment is based on the simple idea that living healthy is fundamentally valuable. I'm not talking about fewer doctor bills or increased productivity at work, but about how you want to experience the rest of your life.

Everyone agrees that health is the single most valuable thing you have. It is the stuff from which everything else—love, success, friends, work satisfaction—is made. Yet I am constantly amazed that so many people choose to spend the time they have on earth feeling tired and irritable, pressured and under the gun. Many of my patients had become used to feeling less than well, used to living with chronic physical and psychological problems, used to lacking the energy to function at their best true level.

They were so accustomed to "non-health" that they forgot they had a choice. They forgot that they can recognize the factors that shape our well-being and *do something about it*.

You now know that the Immune Power Diet is not like many other diet plans, a series of "don'ts" based on depriving your body, undermining its biochemistry and integrity.

On the contrary, my nutrition plan accentuates the positive, putting every area of your nutrition on your side in order to help you build up your body's own spectacularly efficient health system.

In addition, this program is based on the state-of-the-art medical research. The findings I have cited throughout the book are consistent with the best scientific information available in the world today.

Does that mean this is the ultimate nutritional program? No—there's no such thing. This field is changing and growing so rapidly, and we are learning so much so fast, that we are far from having any ultimate answers. It is no wonder much of this book may seem controversial because we still have so much to learn about preventive, immune nutrition. Discoveries are being made at an amazing pace. Students in the most innovative medical schools are studying preventive immunology as a core part of medical education. I have absolutely no doubt that in ten years the concepts in this book will be generally accepted by the medical community.

But you don't have to wait for a decade—I want to make sure that you can put that knowledge to work *right now* in your life to renew and rebuild every area of your health, energy, and appearance.

DON'T FORGET . . .

There are two especially important points to remember as you put Immune Power to work:

- You may have withdrawal symptoms during the first week or so of the diet. These are nothing to worry about—in fact, they are positive proof that the diet is working. If this is a problem for you, go back and re-read the advice in chapter 3.
- If you take some medication regularly or are under a doctor's care for chronic illness, you may notice changes in the effectiveness of your medicine as your "immune tune" improves. As you lose weight and get healthier, you may find that less medicine works just as well. You should always inform your physician if you are on the Immune Power Diet program, so that you can be monitored for these kinds of changes.

WHAT DO YOU HAVE TO GIVE UP?

I won't deny that the Immune Power Diet asks you to make some real changes in how you look at food, but I am not asking you to become a food Puritan. All you must do is identify and then eliminate the hidden toxins which are now damaging your health and energy. Once your body has recovered from the effect of those hidden food sensitivities, you can eat them again on a moderate schedule. You will find very few foods that have to be totally cut out of your life. Of course, there may be foods that you decide to avoid permanently because *you* decide they produce such strong unpleasant reactions.

CHOOSE THE PROGRAM YOU NEED

IF YOUR FIRST INTEREST IS WEIGHT LOSS

Those of you for whom weight loss is a key ingredient to improved health—those who need to lose twenty, thirty, or even sixty pounds—will want to start with the Elimination Diet in section II. There, you will find the safest most effective way to shed those pounds that keep you unhealthy.

But your program doesn't stop there. After you have experienced the dramatic weight loss that diet can bring, you will further benefit from raising your Immune Quotient, as described in Section II. (You will also want to enjoy the recipes in Section II to help you maintain your weight loss and improved health.) To get the most out of this book, follow the diet in section II, rebuilding immune health in section III, and the maintenance recipes in section II.

IF YOUR FIRST INTEREST IS HEALTH AND VITALITY

Are you mainly interested in the wide-ranging health benefits of Immune Power? If you are now at your ideal weight, your main goal is obviously not weight loss. You have come to this diet to improve your health, longevity, energy, vitality, and the quality of your life.

Of course, even if you are one of the lucky ones who have no problem with excess weight, you aren't necessarily healthy. There are scores of other variables affecting your health: your cardiac profile, cholesterol level, blood pressure, sedementation rate (a medical test which is an overall index of illness), and many others.

In my practice I often see patients who are thin, sometimes even too thin, who desperately need to rebuild their immune system. If this is you, your program will focus on identifying hidden food sensitivities (Section II) and improving your Immune Quotient in section III. You will also benefit from using the immune health recipes in section II.

PROMISE YOURSELF: A FAIR TRY

Whatever your goal, you must give the Immune Power Diet program a fair try. Experience with thousands of patients has proved that getting started is the only real hurdle. If you can make a contract with yourself to do that, everything else will follow.

How can I be so sure? Because I have seen over and over again how well this program works. If you try it, you'll like it, as simple as that!

You simply have no idea of how terrific you can feel when your immune power is at its fullest reach.

But, in the words of Confucius, the longest journey begins with a single step. If you are ready to take that step on the road to superb health, you have made your commitment to Immune Power—for life.

Only you can control your immune health so that its power works for you. I wrote this book to give you the opportunity to use the most current technology and information immediately so that you may truly treat yourself most effectively. Please start now!

Index

ABOUT THE AUTHOR

STUART M. BERGER, M.D., received his medical degree from Tufts University and pursued research at the Harvard School of Public Health, studying the effects of nutrition and psychology on weight control. He is the author of the bestselling *The Southampton Diet* and has a prestigious practice in Manhattan, where his patients include some of the most famous and powerful figures of our time.

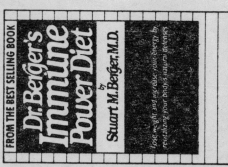